# ABC of

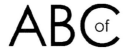

# COPD

## Third Edition

EDITED BY

*Graeme P. Currie*

Aberdeen Royal Infirmary
Aberdeen, UK

**WILEY** Blackwell

BMJ Books

*Registered Offices*
John Wiley & Sons, Inc., 111 River Street, Hoboken, NJ 07030, USA
John Wiley & Sons Ltd, The Atrium, Southern Gate, Chichester, West Sussex, PO19 8SQ, UK

*Editorial Office*
9600 Garsington Road, Oxford, OX4 2DQ, UK
For details of our global editorial offices, customer services, and more information about Wiley products visit us at www.wiley.com.

Wiley also publishes its books in a variety of electronic formats and by print-on-demand. Some content that appears in standard print versions of this book may not be available in other formats.

*Library of Congress Cataloging-in-Publication Data*

Name: Currie, Graeme P., editor.
Title: ABC of COPD / [edited] by Dr Graeme P. Currie.
Description: Third edition. | Hoboken, NJ : Wiley, 2017. | Series: ABC series | Includes index. |
Identifiers: LCCN 2017014503 (print) | LCCN 2017015850 (ebook) | ISBN 9781119212805 (pdf) |
    ISBN 9781119212812 (epub) | ISBN 9781119212850 (pbk.)
Subjects: | MESH: Pulmonary Disease, Chronic Obstructive
Classification: LCC RC776.O3 (ebook) | LCC RC776.O3 (print) | NLM WF 600 | DDC 616.2/4–dc23
LC record available at https://lccn.loc.gov/2017014503

Cover design: Wiley
Cover image: © gmutlu/Gettyimages

Set in 9.25/12pt Minion by SPi Global, Pondicherry, India
Printed and bound in Singapore by Markono Print Media Pte Ltd

10  9  8  7  6  5  4  3  2  1

ABC of
**COPD**

**Third Edition**

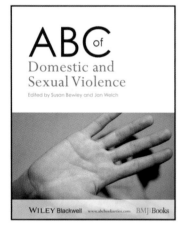
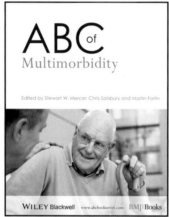
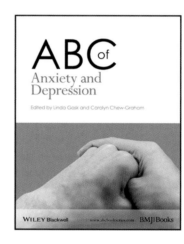
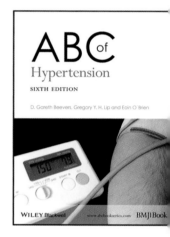
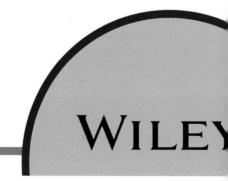

# Contents

# Contributors

**Sanjay Agrawal**

Consultant in Respiratory and Intensive Care Medicine
Respiratory Biomedical Research Unit
Institute of Lung Health
Glenfield Hospital, Leicester, UK

**Peter J. Barnes**

Margaret Turner-Warwick Professor of Medicine
Head of Respiratory Medicine
Airway Disease Section
National Heart and Lung Institute
Imperial College
London, UK

**John R. Britton**

Professor of Epidemiology
UK Centre for Tobacco Control Studies
University of Nottingham;
Consultant in RespiratoryMedicine
City Hospital
Nottingham, UK

**Mahendran Chetty**

Consultant in Respiratory Medicine
Chest Clinic C, Aberdeen Royal Infirmary
Aberdeen, Scotland, UK

**Graeme P. Currie**

Consultant in Respiratory Medicine
Chest Clinic C, Aberdeen Royal Infirmary
Aberdeen, Scotland, UK

**Graham S. Devereux**

Consultant in Respiratory Medicine
Chest Clinic C, Aberdeen Royal Infirmary
Aberdeen, Scotland, UK

**Graham Douglas**

Retired Consultant in Respiratory Medicine
Chest Clinic C, Aberdeen Royal Infirmary
Aberdeen, Scotland, UK

**Claire Fotheringham**

Principal Clinical Respiratory Physiologist
Pulmonary Function Department
Aberdeen Royal Infirmary
Aberdeen, Scotland, UK

**Cathy Jackson**

Head of School
School of Medicine
University of Central Lancashire
Preston, UK

**Gordon Linklater**

Consultant in Palliative Medicine
Highland Hospice
Inverness, Scotland, UK

**Brian J. Lipworth**

Consultant in Respiratory Medicine
Scottish Centre for Respiratory Research
Ninewells Hospital and Medical School
Dundee, Scotland, UK

**James L. Lordan**

Consultant Respiratory and Lung Transplant Physician
Freeman Hospital
University of Newcastle-upon-Tyne
Newcastle-upon-Tyne, UK

**Margaret Macleod**

Senior Respiratory Physiotherapist
Chest Clinic C, Aberdeen Royal Infirmary
Aberdeen, Scotland, UK

**William MacNee**

Professor of Respiratory and Environmental Medicine
MRC Centre for Inflammation Research
Queen's Medical Research Institute
University of Edinburgh
Edinburgh, Scotland, UK

**David R. Miller**
Consultant in Respiratory Medicine
Chest Clinic C, Aberdeen Royal Infirmary
Aberdeen, Scotland, UK

**Paul K. Plant**
Consultant Chest Physician and Clinical Director
for Respiratory Services
North Cumbria University Hospitals NHS Trust
Carlisle, UK

**Roberto A. Rabinovich**
Senior Clinical Research Fellow
MRC Centre for Inflammation Research
Queen's Medical Research Institute
University of Edinburgh
Edinburgh, Scotland, UK

**Morag Reilly**
Primary Care Respiratory Nurse
Aberdeen City Health and Social Care Community Partnership
Aberdeen, Scotland, UK

**Waleed Salih**
Specialist Registrar in Respiratory Medicine
Ninewells Hospital and Medical School
Dundee, Scotland, UK

**Stuart Schembri**
Consultant in Respiratory Medicine
Ninewells Hospital and Medical School
Dundee, Scotland, UK

**Stephen Stott**
Consultant Intensivist
Aberdeen Royal Infirmary
Aberdeen, Scotland, UK

# Foreword

Chronic obstructive pulmonary disease (COPD) continues to be a major global health problem. It is the fourth most common cause of death globally, and in industrialised countries like the UK, has now risen to the third most common cause of death. In the UK, the mortality from COPD in women now well exceeds that of breast cancer. COPD is also the fifth most common cause of chronic disability, increasing because of more prevalent cigarette smoking in developing countries and, most importantly, because of a rapidly ageing population. COPD now affects approximately 10% of individuals over 40 years and is equally common in women, reflecting the lack of gender difference in smoking. Acute exacerbations of COPD remain one of the most common causes of hospital admission. Because of this, COPD has an increasing economic impact, and healthcare costs now exceed those of asthma many times.

Despite these startling statistics, COPD has been relatively neglected and is still greatly underdiagnosed in general practice, where spirometry, needed to establish the diagnosis, is still very underused. This is in marked contrast to asthma which is now recognised and well managed in the community.

There are highly effective medications available for asthma which have transformed patients' lives. Sadly, this is not the case in COPD where treatments are less effective while no treatment has so far been shown to slow the relentless progression of the disease. However, important advances have been made in understanding the underlying disease and in managing patients with COPD. Of particular importance has been the introduction of several new long-acting bronchodilators (β-agonists and muscarinic antagonists) and their combinations, which have been found to be the most effective way to reduce symptoms and prevent exacerbations, particularly in those with severe disease.

In this new edition of the ABC series on COPD, Graeme Currie and colleagues provide an update on diagnosis, pathophysiology and modern management of COPD. There have been important advances since the first edition of the book over 10 years ago. Once the disease is recognised, pharmacological and non-pharmacological treatments are able to greatly improve the quality of life of patients with COPD. It is important that COPD is recognised and treated appropriately in general practice where most of these patients are managed and this book provides an easy-to-read overview of the key issues in this important disease.

Peter J. Barnes FRS, FMedSci

# CHAPTER 1

# Definition, Epidemiology and Risk Factors

*Graham S. Devereux*

Division of Applied Health Sciences, University of Aberdeen, Aberdeen, UK
Aberdeen Royal Infirmary, Aberdeen, UK

---

**OVERVIEW**

- Chronic obstructive pulmonary disease (COPD) is defined by relatively fixed airflow obstruction.
- The number of individuals diagnosed with COPD is far less than the actual number thought to be affected. Prevalence increases with age and socioeconomic deprivation.
- Globally, COPD is projected to be the third leading cause of death by 2030 with the majority of deaths likely to be in low-/middle-income countries.
- The impact of COPD, particularly exacerbations, on health service resource is considerable.
- Risk factors for COPD include cigarette smoking, indoor air pollution (particularly close and regular exposure to combustion of biomass fuels), outdoor air pollution, occupational exposure to some dusts, vapours, irritants and fumes and α1-antitrypsin deficiency.

---

## Definition

Chronic obstructive pulmonary disease (COPD) is a progressive lung disease characterised by airflow destruction and destruction of the lung parenchyma. The widely used definition put forward by the Global Initiative for Chronic Obstructive Lung Disease (GOLD) is that COPD is 'a common preventable and treatable disease characterised by persistent airflow limitation that is usually progressive and associated with an enhanced chronic inflammatory response in the airways and the lungs to noxious particles or gases. Exacerbations and comorbidities contribute to the overall severity in individual patients'.

COPD is the preferred name for the airflow obstruction associated with the diseases of chronic bronchitis and emphysema (Box 1.1). A number of other conditions are associated with poorly reversible airflow obstruction, for example bronchiectasis and obliterative bronchiolitis. Although these conditions need to be considered in the differential diagnosis of obstructive airways disease, they are not conventionally covered by the definition of COPD. Although asthma is defined by variable airflow obstruction, there is evidence suggesting that the airway remodelling processes associated with asthma can result in irreversible progressive airflow obstruction that fulfils the definition for COPD. Because of the high prevalence of asthma and COPD, these conditions co-exist in a sizeable proportion of individuals and can raise diagnostic uncertainty.

---

Box 1.1 **Definitions of conditions associated with airflow obstruction.**

- COPD is a common preventable and treatable disease characterised by persistent airflow limitation that is usually progressive and associated with an enhanced chronic inflammatory response in the airways and the lung to noxious particles or gases. Exacerbations and co-morbidities contribute to the overall severity in individual patients.
- Chronic bronchitis is defined as the presence of chronic productive cough on most days for 3 months, in each of 2 consecutive years, in a patient whom other causes of productive cough have been excluded.
- Emphysema is defined as abnormal, permanent enlargement of the distal airspaces, distal to the terminal bronchioles, accompanied by destruction of their walls and without obvious fibrosis.
- Asthma is characterised by widespread narrowing of the bronchial airways which changes in severity over short periods of time, either spontaneously or following treatment.

---

## Epidemiology

### Prevalence

The prevalence of COPD varies considerably between epidemiological surveys. While this reflects the variation between and within countries, differences in methodology, diagnostic criteria and analytical techniques undoubtedly contribute to disparities among studies. There is no consensus as to the optimal metric of COPD prevalence. The lower estimates of prevalence are usually

---

*ABC of COPD*, Third Edition. Edited by Graeme P. Currie.
© 2017 John Wiley & Sons Ltd. Published 2017 by John Wiley & Sons Ltd.

based on self-reported or 'doctor-confirmed' COPD and are typically 40–50% of the rates derived when spirometry is used. The underdiagnosis of COPD probably arises because many individuals fail to recognise the significance of symptoms and present relatively late with moderate or severe airflow obstruction (Figures 1.1–1.3).

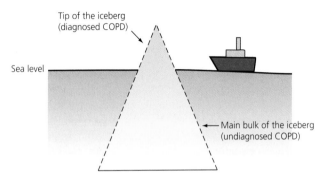

**Figure 1.1** Known cases of COPD may represent only the 'tip of the iceberg' with many cases currently undiagnosed.

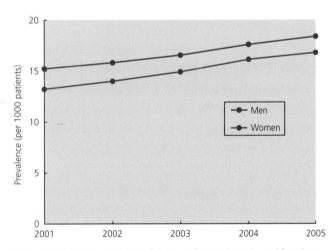

**Figure 1.2** Lifetime prevalence of diagnosed COPD in males and females (per 1000) resident in England 2001–2005. Figure adapted from Simpson CR, Hippisley-Cox J, Sheikh A. Trends in the epidemiology of chronic obstructive pulmonary disease in England: a national study of 51 804 patients. *British Journal of General Practice* 2010; **60**(576): 277–284.

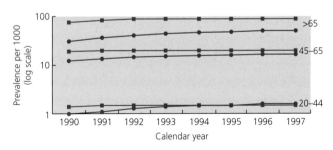

**Figure 1.3** Prevalence (per 1000) of diagnosed COPD in UK men (■) and women (●) grouped by age, between 1990 and 1997. Reproduced from Soriano JB, Maier WC, Egger P et al. *Thorax* 2000; **55**: 789–794, with permission of BMJ Publishing Group.

Globally, the World Health Organization (WHO) estimates that 65 million people have moderate to severe COPD. In the UK, a national study reported that 10% of males and 11% of females aged 16–65 had an abnormally low $FEV_1$. Similarly, in Manchester, non-reversible airflow obstruction was present in 11% of subjects aged >45 years, of whom 65% had not been diagnosed with COPD. In the UK, an estimated 3 million individuals have COPD but only 1.2 million have a formal diagnosis. In the US, an estimated 24 million have evidence of impaired lung function consistent with COPD, while 12.7 million US adults have diagnosed disease. In a study of 12 countries in Europe, North America, China, Australia, South Africa and the Philippines, the prevalence of COPD in those over the age of 40 years based on lung function criteria was 10.1%, being more common in males (11.8%) than females (8.5%). The prevalence of COPD increases with age, almost doubling with each decade from the age of 40 years. In the UK, the lifetime prevalence of diagnosed COPD has been reported to be increasing and is more common in males than females. In contrast, in the US the prevalence of COPD has been reported to be stable, with the disease being more common in females. COPD is associated with socioeconomic deprivation. In a systematic review, individuals from the lowest socioeconomic strata were at least twice as likely to have COPD when compared with more affluent individuals, regardless of the population studied, metric of socioeconomic status or COPD outcome investigated (Figures 1.4, 1.5).

## Mortality

Globally, COPD was ranked sixth as the cause of death in 1990, but with the ageing of the world population, the epidemic of cigarette smoking in developing countries and reduced mortality from other currently common causes of death (e.g. ischaemic heart disease and infectious diseases), it is expected that COPD will become the third leading cause of death worldwide by 2030. In 2012, an estimated 6%

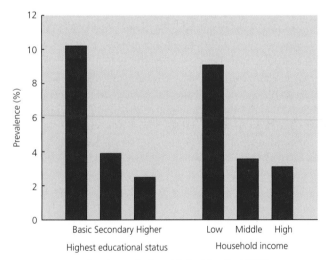

Prevalence of spirometrically determined COPD in a Finnish National Survey

**Figure 1.4** Prevalence of COPD confirmed by spirometry in a Finnish National Survey: association with metrics of socioeconomic status. Figure derived using data from Kanervisto M et al. Low socioeconomic status is associated with chronic obstructive airway diseases. *Respiratory Medicine* 2011; **105**: 1140–1146.

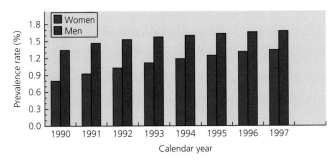

**Figure 1.5** Prevalence of diagnosed COPD in UK men and women (per 1000) between 1990 and 1997. Reproduced from Soriano JB, Maier WC, Egger P et al. *Thorax* 2000; **55**: 789–794, with permission of BMJ Publishing Group.

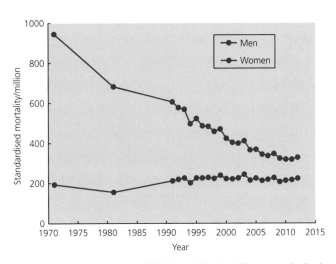

**Figure 1.6** UK death rates from COPD since 1971. Mortality age-standardised rates per million. based on the European Standard Population. Figure derived using data from death registrations, selected data tables, England and Wales 2013. Office for National Statistics, London. www.ons.gov.uk/ons/datasets-and-tables/index.html?pageSize=50&sortBy=none&sortDirection=none&newquery=standardised+mortality+by+cause+and+age+DR+series.

(3 million) of deaths worldwide were attributed to COPD, and more than 90% of these occurred in low- and middle-income countries. In the UK in 2014, there were approximately 30 000 deaths attributed to COPD, with 15 300 of these deaths in males and 14 700 in females. These figures suggest that in the UK, COPD underlies 5.3% of all deaths, 5.5% of male deaths and 5.0% of female deaths. In the US, the most recent data, covering 1999–2013, indicate that 136 000 (5.5%) deaths are a consequence of COPD, and that it is the third leading cause of death behind cancer and heart disease.

In the UK, over the last 40 years, mortality rates due to COPD have fallen in males and risen in females. In the US, the age-adjusted death rate for COPD in males is approximately 1.3 times greater than the rate in females. However, since there are more females in the general US population than males, the actual number of females dying from COPD has exceeded the number of males dying since about 1999. COPD mortality rates increase with age, disease severity and socioeconomic disadvantage. On average, in the UK COPD reduces life expectancy by 1.8 years (76.5 versus 78.3 years for controls). Mild disease reduces life expectancy by 1.1 years, moderate disease by 1.7 years and severe disease by 4.1 years. In the US, it has been estimated that a male smoker at the age of 65 years will have his life expectancy reduced by 0.3, 2.2 and 5.8 years, with mild, moderate and severe disease respectively. For a female smoker at age 65, mild, moderate and severe COPD is associated with reduced life expectancies of 0.2, 2.0 and 6.1 years respectively (Figure 1.6).

## Morbidity and economic impact

The morbidity and economic costs associated with COPD are very high, generally unrecognised and more than twice those associated with asthma. The impact on quality of life is particularly high in patients with frequent exacerbations, although even patients with mild COPD have an impaired quality of life.

In the UK, emergency hospital admissions for COPD have steadily increased as a percentage of all admissions, from 0.5% in 1991 to 1% in 2000 and 1.5% in 2008–2009. In 2008–2009, COPD exacerbations resulted in 164 000 hospital admissions in the UK, with an average duration of stay of 7.8 days, accounting for 1.3 million bed-days. COPD is the second largest cause of emergency admission to hospital in the UK and is one of the most costly inpatient conditions treated by the National Health Service (NHS). At least 10% of emergency admissions to hospital are as a consequence of COPD

and this proportion is even greater during the winter. Approximately 25% of individuals diagnosed with COPD are admitted to hospital and about 15% of all patients are admitted each year. In the US in 2010, there were an estimated 715 000 hospital discharges with COPD as the first-listed condition, while in contrast to the UK, the number and rate of COPD hospitalizations remained unchanged between 1999 and 2010. In both the US and the UK, there has been an increase in the proportion of COPD admissions that are female. In the UK, similar proportions of males and females are admitted with exacerbations of COPD, but in the US since 1993 COPD discharge rates for females have been higher than for males.

The impact in primary care is even greater in that 86% of care is exclusively provided by primary care. It has been estimated that an average general practitioner's list will include 200 patients with COPD (even more in areas of social deprivation), although not all will be diagnosed. It has also been estimated that COPD is responsible for 1.4 million GP consultations annually and that each diagnosed patient costs the UK economy £1639 each year, equating to a national burden of £982 million. For each patient, annual direct costs to the NHS are £819, with 54% of this due to hospital admissions and 19% due to drug treatment. COPD has further societal costs: about 40% of UK patients are below retirement age and the disease prevents about 25% from working and reduces the capacity to work in a further 10%. Annual indirect costs of COPD have been estimated at £820 per patient and consist of the costs of disability, absence from work, premature mortality and the time caregivers miss work. Within Europe, it has been estimated that in 2001, the overall cost of COPD to the European economy was €38.7 billion (€4.7 billion for ambulatory care, €2.7 billion for drugs, €2.9 billion for inpatient care and €28.4 billion for lost working days). In the US, the National Heart Lung and Blood Institute estimated that the national annual cost to the US economy of COPD in 2010 was $49.9 billion ($29.5 billion in direct healthcare expenditure, $8.0 billion in lost productivity and $12.4 billion in lost productivity attributable to premature deaths) (Figures 1.7–1.9).

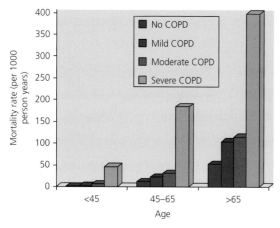

**Figure 1.7** UK deaths from COPD (per 1000 person-years) by age and severity of COPD. Figure derived using data from Soriano JB, Maier WC, Egger P et al. *Thorax* 2000; **55**: 789–794. Reproduced with permission of BMJ Publishing Group.

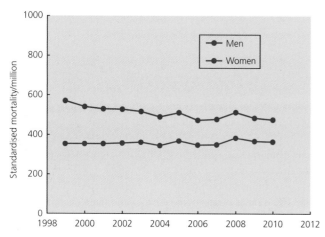

**Figure 1.8** COPD mortality in the United States of America, 1999–2010, expressed as standardised mortality per million. Figure redrawn with data from www.cdc.gov/copd/pdfs/graph_copd_death_rates_united_states1999_2010.pdf.

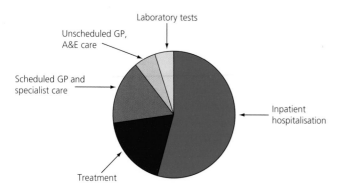

**Figure 1.9** An analysis of the direct costs of COPD to the NHS. A&E, accident and emergency; GP, general practitioner. Figure derived with data from Britton M. The burden of COPD in the UK: results from the Confronting COPD survey. *Respiratory Medicine* 2003; **97**(suppl C): S71–S79.

## Risk factors

### Smoking

In developed countries, cigarette smoking is the single most important risk factor in the development of COPD, with studies consistently reporting dose–response associations and accelerated decline

in lung function. Current smoking is also associated with an increased diagnosis and death. Pipe and cigar smokers have significantly greater morbidity and mortality from COPD than non-smokers, although the risk is less than for cigarettes. Approximately 50% of cigarette smokers develop airflow obstruction and 10–20% develop clinically significant COPD. The risk of developing lung function evidence of COPD increases by 20% for each 10 pack-years of smoking. Although smoking is the dominant risk factor, it is not a prerequisite. It is now increasingly apparent that 5–12% of people with diagnosed COPD have never smoked and based on spirometry, 20–40% of individuals with COPD have either never smoked or have a minimal cumulative smoking history.

Maternal smoking during and after pregnancy is associated with reduced infant, childhood and adult lung function, days, weeks and years after birth respectively. Most studies have demonstrated that the effects of antenatal environmental tobacco smoking exposure are greater in magnitude and independent of associations with postnatal exposure.

## Other factors

An increasing number of risk factors other than smoking have been associated with COPD, particularly in developing countries (Box 1.2). These non-smoking risk factors include indoor (biomass) and outdoor air pollution, occupational exposures and early life factors such as intrauterine growth retardation, poor nutrition, repeated lower respiratory tract infections and a history of pulmonary tuberculosis.

Box 1.2 **Non-smoking risk factors associated with the development of COPD.**

*Indoor air pollution*
- Smoke from biomass fuel: plant residues (wood, charcoal, crops, twigs, dried grass) animal residues (dung)
- Smoke from coal

*Occupational exposures*
- Crop farming: grain dust, organic dust, inorganic dust
- Animal farming: organic dust, ammonia, hydrogen sulphide
- Dust exposures: coal mining, hard rock mining, tunnelling, concrete manufacture, construction, brick manufacture, gold mining, iron and steel founding
- Chemical exposures: plastic, textile, rubber industries, leather manufacture, manufacture of food products
- Pollutant exposure: transportation and trucking, automotive repair

*Treated pulmonary tuberculosis*
*Repeated childhood lower respiratory tract infections*
*Chronic asthma*
*Outdoor air pollution*
- Particulate matter (<10 μm or <2.5 μm diameter)
- Nitrogen dioxide
- Carbon monoxide

*Poor socioeconomic status*
*Low educational attainment*
*Poor nutrition*

Reproduced with permission from Salvi SS, Barnes PJ. Chronic obstructive pulmonary disease in non-smokers. *Lancet* 2009; **374**: 733–743.

Many of these risk factors are interrelated; for example, biomass smoke exposure is associated with intrauterine growth retardation and repeated early life lower respiratory tract infections.

## Air pollution

Urban air pollution may be involved in lung function development and consequently be a risk factor for COPD. Cross-sectional studies have demonstrated that higher levels of atmospheric air pollution are associated with cough, sputum production, breathlessness and reduced lung function. Exposure to particulate and nitrogen dioxide air pollution has been associated with impaired lung function in adults and reduced lung growth in children.

Worldwide, approximately 3 billion individuals are exposed to indoor air pollution from burning biomass fuel (wood, charcoal, animal waste) in open fires or poorly functioning stoves for cooking and heating. It has been estimated that biomass smoke exposure underlies about 50% of COPD in developing countries. Exposure to biomass smoke is a particular problem for females and young children who are heavily exposed during food preparation. Exposure to biomass smoke has been reported to increase the risk of COPD 2–3-fold.

## Occupation

Some occupational environments with intense prolonged exposure to irritating dusts, gases and fumes can cause COPD independently of cigarette smoking. However, smoking appears to enhance the effects of occupational exposure by increasing the risk of COPD development. It has been estimated that about 15–20% of diagnosed cases are attributable to occupation, and in life-long non-smokers this proportion increases to about 30%. Occupations that have been associated with a higher prevalence of COPD include coal mining, hard rock mining, tunnel working, concrete manufacture, construction, farming, foundry working, the manufacture of plastics, textiles, rubber, leather and food products, transportation and trucking (Figure 1.10) The increasing recognition that occupation can contribute to the development of COPD emphasises the importance of taking a full chronological occupational history.

## α1-Antitrypsin deficiency

The best documented genetic risk factor for COPD is α1-antitrypsin deficiency. However, this is rare and is present in only 1–2% of patients with COPD. α1-Antitrypsin is a glycoprotein responsible for the majority of antiprotease activity in serum. The α1-antitrypsin gene is highly polymorphic, although some genotypes (usually ZZ) are associated with low serum levels. Severe deficiency of α1-antitrypsin is associated with premature and accelerated development of COPD in smokers and non-smokers, although the rate of decline is accelerated in those who smoke. The α1-antitrypsin status of patients with severe COPD who are less than 40 years of age should be determined since over 50% have α1-antitrypsin deficiency. The detection of such cases identifies family members who require genetic counselling and patients who might be suitable for future potential treatment with α1-antitrypsin replacement or lung transplantation.

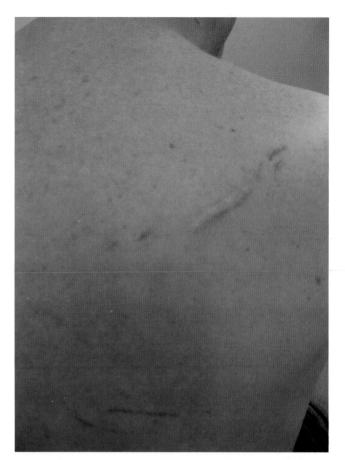

**Figure 1.10** This patient (with minimal smoking history) was found to have chronic obstructive pulmonary disease, with his occupation (coal miner) being the main risk factor. The image shows coal dust tattoos on his back.

## Further reading

American Lung Association. Trends in COPD (Chronic Bronchitis and Emphysema): Morbidity and Mortality. Available at: www.lung.org/assets/documents/research/copd-trend-report.pdf (accessed 20 February 2017).

Britton M. The burden of COPD in the UK: results from the Confronting COPD survey. *Respiratory Medicine* 2003; **97**(suppl C): S71–S79.

Buist AS, McBurnie MA, Vollmer WM et al. International variation in the prevalence of COPD (The BOLD Study): a population-based prevalence study. *Lancet* 2007; **370**: 741–750.

Gershon AS, Dolmage TE, Stephenson A, Jackson B. Chronic obstructive pulmonary disease and socioeconomic status: a systematic review. *Journal of COPD* 2012; **9**: 216–226.

Global Initiative for Chronic Obstructive Lung Disease (GOLD). Global Strategy for the Diagnosis, Management and Prevention of COPD. Available at: http://goldcopd.org/gold-2017-global-strategy-diagnosis-management-prevention-copd/ (accessed 20 February 2017).

Pride NB, Soriano JB. Chronic obstructive pulmonary disease in the United Kingdom: trends in mortality, morbidity and smoking. *Current Opinion in Pulmonary Medicine* 2002; **8**: 95–101.

Salvi SS, Barnes PJ. Chronic obstructive pulmonary disease in non-smokers. *Lancet* 2009; **374**: 733–743.

# CHAPTER 2

# Pathology and Pathogenesis

*William MacNee and Roberto A. Rabinovich*

MRC Centre for Inflammation Research, Queen's Medical Research Institute, University of Edinburgh, Edinburgh, UK

## OVERVIEW

- The clinical sequelae of chronic obstructive pulmonary disease (COPD) result from pathological changes in the large airways (bronchitis), small airways (bronchiolitis) and alveolar space (emphysema).

- Combinations of pathological changes occur to varying degrees in different individuals.

- Chronic inflammation, involving neutrophils, macrophages and T-lymphocytes, is found in the airways and alveolar space.

- Small airway inflammation (bronchiolitis) can lead eventually to scarring; this important pathological change is difficult to assess by conventional lung function tests, but is a major source of airway obstruction.

- In COPD, lungs show an amplified and persistent inflammatory response following exposure to particles, fumes and gases, particularly those found in cigarette smoke.

## Introduction

Chronic obstructive pulmonary disease (COPD) is characterized by persistent airflow limitation. This is usually progressive and associated with an enhanced chronic inflammatory response in the airways and the lung to noxious particles or gases. The latter represents the innate and adaptive immune responses to a lifetime of exposure to noxious particles, fumes and gases, particularly cigarette smoke. All cigarette smokers have inflammatory changes within their lungs, but those who develop COPD exhibit an enhanced or abnormal inflammatory response to inhaled toxic agents. This amplified inflammatory response may result in mucous hypersecretion (chronic bronchitis), tissue destruction (emphysema), disruption of normal repair and defence mechanisms causing small airway inflammation (bronchiolitis) and fibrosis.

In general, the inflammatory and structural changes in the lungs persist on smoking cessation and become more pronounced as the severity of airflow limitation increases. These pathological changes result in increased resistance to airflow in the small conducting airways, increased compliance and reduced elastic recoil of the lungs. This causes progressive airflow limitation and air trapping, which represent the hallmark features of COPD. There is increasing

understanding of the cellular and molecular mechanisms that result in the pathological changes found and how these lead to physiological abnormalities and subsequent development of symptoms. COPD can develop in never smokers but characteristics of lung inflammation in these individuals are not well described.

## Pathology

Pathological changes in the lungs of patients with COPD are found in the proximal and peripheral airways, lung parenchyma and pulmonary vasculature. These changes are present to different extents in affected individuals (Box 2.1, Figures 2.1–2.3).

---

Box 2.1 **Pathological changes found in COPD.**

**Proximal airways (cartilaginous airways >2 mm in diameter)**
- ↑ Macrophages and CD8 T-lymphocytes
- Few neutrophils and eosinophils (neutrophils increase with progressive disease)
- Submucosal bronchial gland enlargement and goblet cell metaplasia (results in excessive mucous production or chronic bronchitis)
- Cellular infiltrates (neutrophils and lymphocytes) of bronchial glands
- Airway epithelial squamous metaplasia, ciliary dysfunction, ↑ smooth muscle and connective tissue

**Peripheral airways (non-cartilaginous airways >2 mm diameter)**
- Bronchiolitis at an early stage
- ↑ Macrophages and T-lymphocytes (CD8 > CD4)
- Few neutrophils or eosinophils
- Pathological extension of goblet cells and squamous metaplasia into peripheral airways
- Luminal and inflammatory exudates
- ↑ B-lymphocytes, lymphoid follicles and fibroblasts
- Peribronchial fibrosis and airway narrowing with progressive disease

**Lung parenchyma (respiratory bronchioles and alveoli)**
- ↑ Macrophages and CD8 T-lymphocytes
- Alveolar wall destruction due to loss of epithelial and endothelial cells
- Development of emphysema (abnormal enlargement of airspaces distal to terminal bronchioles)

---

*ABC of COPD*, Third Edition. Edited by Graeme P. Currie.

- Microscopic emphysematous changes:
  - centrilobular (dilatation and destruction of respiratory bronchioles – commonly found in smokers and predominantly in upper zones)
  - panacinar (destruction of the whole acinus – commonly found in α1-antitrypsin deficiency and more common in lower zones)
- Macroscopic emphysematous changes: microscopic changes progress to bullae formation (defined as an emphysematous airspace >1 cm in diameter)

### Pulmonary vasculature
- ↑ Macrophages and T-lymphocytes
- Early changes:
  - intimal thickening
  - endothelial dysfunction
- Late changes:
  - ↑ vascular smooth muscle
  - collagen deposition
  - destruction of capillary bed
  - development of pulmonary hypertension and cor pulmonale

## Pathogenesis

### Exposure to cigarette smoking, fumes, gases and particles

Cigarette smoking is the major risk factor for COPD, although it is recognised in never smokers, especially in less well-developed countries. In individuals with similar smoking histories (in terms of pack-years), not all will develop COPD due to differences in genetic predisposition to the disease. Exposure to particles and fumes in the workplace from ambient air pollution or the burning of biomass fuel for heating or cooking are also risk factors.

Inflammation is present in the lungs, particularly in the small airways, of all smokers. This normal protective response to inhaled toxins is amplified in COPD and persists even after smoking cessation by mechanisms that are not fully understood. Oxidative stress and an excess of proteinases in the lung modify the lung inflammation and lead to tissue destruction, impairment of defence mechanisms that limit such destruction and disruption of repair mechanisms. A number of mechanisms have been considered to be

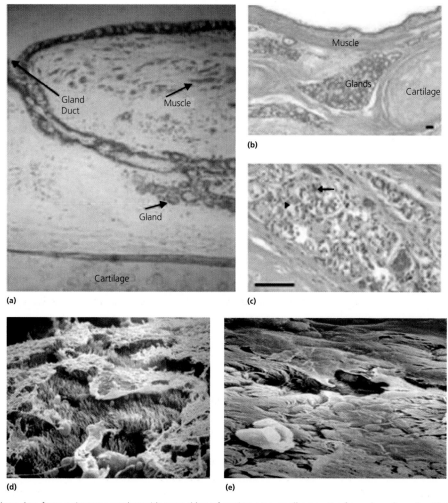

(a)

(b)

(c)

(d)

(e)

**Figure 2.1** (a) A central bronchus from a cigarette smoker with normal lung function. Very small amounts of muscle and small epithelial glands are shown. (b) Bronchial wall from a patient with chronic bronchitis showing a thick bundle of muscle and enlarged glands. (c) A higher magnification of the enlarged glands from (b) showing chronic inflammation involving polymorphonuclear (*arrowhead*) and mononuclear cells, including plasma cells (*arrow*). Printed with kind permission from J.C. Hogg and S. Green. (d) Scanning electron micrograph of airway from a normal individual showing flakes of mucus overlying the cilia. (e) Scanning electron micrograph of a bronchial wall in a patient with chronic bronchitis. Cilia are covered with a blanket of mucus.

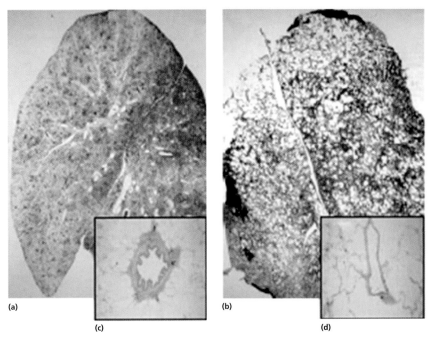

**Figure 2.2** (a) Paper-mounted whole lung section of a normal lung. (b) Paper-mounted whole lung section from a lung with severe centrilobular emphysema. Note that the centrilobular form is more extensive in the upper regions of the lung. (c) Histological section of a normal small airway and surrounding alveoli connecting with attached alveolar walls. (d) Histological section showing emphysema with enlarged alveolar spaces, loss of alveolar walls and alveolar attachments and collapsed airway.

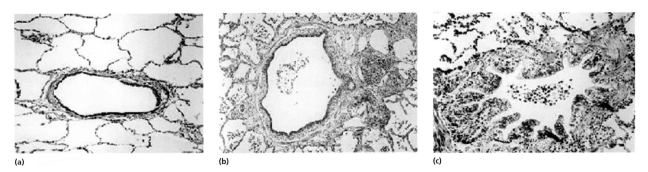

**Figure 2.3** Histological sections of peripheral airways. (a) Section from a cigarette smoker with normal lung function showing a nearly normal airway with small numbers of inflammatory cells. (b) Section from a patient with small airway disease showing inflammatory exudate in the wall and lumen of the airway. (c) Section showing more advanced small airway disease, with reduced lumen causing structural reorganisation of the airway wall, increased smooth muscle and deposition of peribronchial connective tissue. Images produced with kind permission of Professor James C. Hogg, University of British Columbia, Canada.

involved in intensifying lung inflammation, which results in the pathological changes in COPD (Figure 2.4).

## Genetics

There is a significant familial risk of airflow limitation in smoking siblings of patients with severe COPD, suggesting that genetics together with environmental factors influence the susceptibility to COPD. The best documented genetic risk factor is a severe hereditary deficiency of α1-antitrypsin, a major circulating inhibitor of serine proteases. The genetic defect PIZZ leads to deficiency of this protease inhibitor, resulting in early-onset COPD when associated particularly with smoking. This illustrates the interaction between genes and environmental exposures. α1-Antitrypsin deficiency accounts for a small proportion of patients with COPD. Several genome-wide association studies indicate a role of this gene for

other genes such as the α-nicotinic acetylcholine receptor and the hedgehog interacting protein gene.

## Lung growth

Failure to attain maximal lung function, due to factors occurring during gestation and birth, and exposures during childhood and adolescence due to low birth weight, passive smoke exposure or early childhood lung infections represent risk factors for the development of COPD.

## Asthma/bronchial hyperreactivity

Asthma may be a risk factor for the development of COPD. In a longitudinal cohort study, adults with asthma had a 12-fold higher risk of COPD compared to healthy controls. Bronchial hyperresponsiveness has also been shown to be an independent predictor of COPD in population studies.

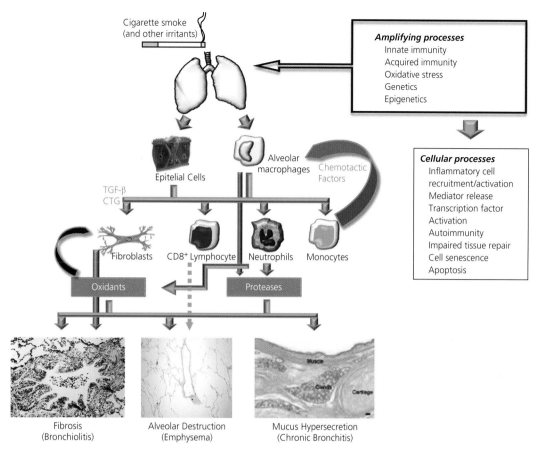

**Figure 2.4** Overview of the pathogenesis of COPD. Cigarette smoke activates macrophages in epithelial cells to produce chemotactic factors that recruit neutrophils and CD8 cells from the circulation. These cells release factors which activate fibroblasts, resulting in abnormal repair processes and bronchiolar fibrosis. An imbalance between proteases released from neutrophils and macrophages and antiproteases leads to alveolar wall destruction (emphysema). Proteases also stimulate the release of mucus. An increased oxidant burden resulting from smoke inhalation or release of oxidants from inflammatory leucocytes causes epithelial and other cells to release chemotactic factors, inactivates antiproteases and directly injures alveolar walls and causes mucus secretion. Several processes are involved in amplifying the inflammatory responses in COPD. TGF-β, transforming growth factor-β; CTG, connective tissue growth factor.

## Chronic bronchitis

Although early studies indicated that chronic bronchitis was not associated with decline in lung function, more recent studies have found an association between mucus hypersecretion and forced expiratory volume in 1 second ($FEV_1$) decline. In younger adults who smoke, the presence of chronic bronchitis is associated with an increased risk of COPD.

## Innate and adaptive immune inflammatory responses

The innate inflammatory immune system provides primary protection against the continuing insult of inhalation of toxic gases, fumes and particles. The first line of defence consists of the mucociliary clearance apparatus and macrophages that clear foreign material from the lower respiratory tract; both of these are impaired in COPD. The second line of defence is the exudation of plasma and circulating cells into both large and small conducting airways and alveoli. This process is controlled by an array of proinflammatory chemokines and cytokines (Box 2.2).

> **Box 2.2 Inflammatory cells and mediators in COPD.**
>
> - Neutrophils – release reactive oxygen species, elastase and cytokines that are involved in the pathogenesis of COPD, with effects on goblet cells, submucosal glands, the induction of emphysema by the release of protease and inflammation. They are increased in the sputum and distal airspaces of smokers; a further increase occurs in COPD and increases with disease severity.
> - Macrophages – produce reactive oxygen species, lipid mediators such as leukotrienes and prostaglandins, cytokines, chemokines and matrix metalloproteases. They are found particularly around small airways and may be associated with both small airway fibrosis and centrilobular emphysema in COPD. They are increased in number in airways, lung parenchyma and bronchoalveolar lavage fluid and increase further with progressive disease severity.
> - Eosinophils – increased numbers of eosinophils have been reported in sputum, bronchoalveolar lavage fluid and the airway wall in some patients with COPD and may represent a distinct subgroup of COPD patients with a good clinical response to corticosteroids.

- T-lymphocytes (CD4 and CD8 cells) – increased in the airways and lung parenchyma with an increase in CD8:CD4 ratio. Numbers of Th1 and Tc1 cells, which produce interferon-γ, also increase. CD8 cells may be cytotoxic from the release of lytic substances such as perforin and granzyme, cause alveolar wall destruction and induce epithelial and endothelial apoptosis.
- B-lymphocytes – increased in the peripheral airways and within lymphoid follicles, possibly as a response to chronic infection or an autoimmune process.

## Inflammatory cells

COPD is characterised by increased neutrophils, macrophages, T-lymphocytes (CD8 > CD4) and dendritic cells in various parts of the lungs (Box 2.2). In general, the extent of inflammation is related to the severity of airflow limitation. These inflammatory cells are capable of releasing a variety of cytokines and mediators which participate in the disease process. This inflammatory cell pattern is markedly different from that found in asthma.

## Inflammatory mediators

Many inflammatory mediators are increased in patients with COPD. These include:

- leukotriene $B_4$ ($LTB_4$), a neutrophil and T-cell chemoattractant, which is produced by macrophages, neutrophils and epithelial cells
- chemotactic factors such as CXC chemokines, interleukin-8 (IL-8) and growth-related oncogene-α produced by macrophages and epithelial cells; these attract cells from the circulation and amplify proinflammatory responses
- proinflammatory cytokines such as tumour necrosis factor-α, IL-1β and IL-6
- growth factors such as transforming growth factor-β (TGF-β), which may cause fibrosis in the airways either directly or through the release of another cytokine (connective tissue growth factor).

An adaptive immune response is also present in the lungs of patients with COPD, as shown by the presence of mature lymphoid follicles. These increase in number in the airways according to disease severity. Their presence has been attributed to the large antigen load associated with bacterial colonisation, frequent lower respiratory tract infections and possibly an autoimmune response that may be involved in the persistence of inflammation after smoking cessation. Dendritic cells are major antigen-presenting cells and are increased in the small airways, and provide a link between innate and adaptive immune responses.

## Protease/antiprotease imbalance

Increased production (or activity) of proteases or inactivation (or reduced production) of antiproteases results in an imbalance that allows the breakdown of connective tissue such as elastin in the alveolar walls that is a feature of emphysema. Cigarette smoke and inflammation *per se* produce oxidative stress, which primes several inflammatory cells to release a combination of proteases and inactivate several antiproteases by oxidation. The major proteases involved in the pathogenesis of COPD are the serine proteases produced by neutrophils, cysteine proteases and matrix metalloproteases (MMPs) produced by macrophages. The major

antiproteases involved in the pathogenesis of emphysema include α1-antitrypsin, secretory leukoproteinase inhibitor and tissue inhibitors of MMP (Box 2.3).

Box 2.3 **Proteinases and antiproteinases involved in COPD.**

| Proteinases | Antiproteinases |
| --- | --- |
| *Serine proteinases* | |
| Neutrophil elastase | α1-Antitrypsin |
| Cathepsin G | Secretory leukoprotease inhibitor |
| Proteinase 3 | Elafin |
| *Cysteine proteinases* | |
| Cathepsins B, K, L, S | Cystatins |
| Matrix metalloproteinases | Tissue inhibitors of MMP |
| (MMP-8, MMP-9, MMP-12) | (TIMP1–4) |

## Oxidative stress

The oxidative burden is increased in COPD. Sources of increased oxidants include cigarette smoke and reactive oxygen and nitrogen species released from inflammatory cells. There is also a reduction in antioxidants as a result of reduction in Nrf2, a transcription factor that regulates many antioxidant genes. This creates an imbalance in oxidants and antioxidants (oxidative stress). Many markers of oxidative stress are increased in stable COPD and are increased further during exacerbations. Oxidative stress can lead to inactivation of antiproteinases and stimulation of mucous production. It can also amplify inflammation by activating many intercellular pathways, including kinases (e.g. P38 mitogen-activated protein (MAP) kinase) enhancing transcription factor activation (e.g. nuclear factor-κB (NF-κB)) and epigenetic events (such as decreasing histone deacetylates) that lead to increased gene expression of proinflammatory mediators.

## Lung microbiome

Polymerase chain reaction (PCR) technology has challenged traditional thinking and demonstrated that the lungs are not a sterile space. Studies suggest that patients with COPD have a distinct lung microbiome (in comparison with healthy individuals) and have increased levels of staphylococci and streptococci, in addition to an outgrowth of Proteobacteria phylum. Changes in the microbiome may have importance in persistent lung inflammation associated with COPD.

## Pathogenesis of emphysema

Emphysema is characterised by enlargement of the airspaces distal to the terminal bronchioles and associated with destruction of alveolar walls but without fibrosis (Box 2.4). Paradoxically, fibrosis may occur in the small airways in COPD. A number of mechanisms are involved in the pathogenesis of emphysema, including protease/antiprotease imbalance, oxidative stress, apoptosis and cell senescence.

Box 2.4 **Mechanism of emphysema in COPD.**

- Protease/antiprotease imbalance – activation of MMPs such as MMP-9 and -12, serine proteases such as neutrophil elastase and inactivation of antiproteases such as α1-antitrypsin
- Activation of CD8 T-cells, which release perforin and granzymes
- Apoptosis of alveolar cells resulting from a decrease in VEGF signalling
- Accelerated lung ageing and cell senescence leading to failure of lung maintenance and repair
- Ineffective clearance of apoptotic cells (efferocytosis) by macrophages, leading to decreased anti-inflammatory mechanisms
- Mitochondrial dysfunction with increased oxidative stress leading to increased cell apoptosis, for example through SIRT-1

MMP, matrix metalloproteinase; SIRT, sirtuin; VEGF, vascular endothelial growth factor.

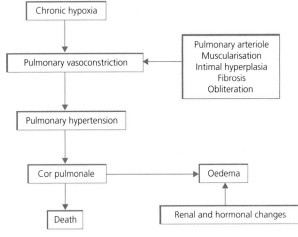

**Figure 2.5** The development of pulmonary hypertension in COPD.

## Pathophysiology

The pathogenic mechanisms described earlier result in the pathological changes found in COPD. These in turn cause physiological abnormalities such as mucous hypersecretion, ciliary dysfunction, airflow limitation and hyperinflation, gas exchange abnormalities, pulmonary hypertension and systemic effects.

### Mucous hypersecretion and ciliary dysfunction

Not all patients with COPD have symptomatic mucus hypersecretion. When present, it is due to an increased number of goblet cells and enlarged submucosal glands in response to chronic airway irritation by cigarette smoke and other noxious agents. Mucous hypersecretion results in a chronic productive cough. This is characteristic of chronic bronchitis, but not necessarily associated with airflow limitation, while not all patients with COPD have symptomatic mucous hypersecretion. Several mediators and proteases stimulate mucus hypersecretion often by way of activation of the epidermal growth factor receptor. Ciliary dysfunction is due to squamous metaplasia of epithelial cells and results in dysfunction of the mucociliary escalator and difficulty expectorating.

### Airflow limitation and hyperinflation/air trapping

Chronic airflow limitation is the physiological hallmark of COPD. The main site of airflow limitation is the small conducting airways that are <2 mm in diameter. This results from inflammation, narrowing (airway remodelling) and inflammatory exudates in the small airways. Other factors contributing to airflow limitation include loss of lung elastic recoil (due to destruction of alveolar walls) and destruction of alveolar support (from alveolar attachments).

The airway obstruction progressively traps air during expiration, resulting in hyperinflation of the lungs at rest and dynamic hyperinflation during exercise. Hyperinflation reduces the inspiratory capacity and, therefore, the functional residual capacity during exercise. These features result in the breathlessness and impaired exercise capacity typical of COPD.

### Gas exchange abnormalities

Gas exchange abnormalities occur in advanced disease and are characterised by arterial hypoxaemia with or without hypercapnia. An abnormal distribution of ventilation/perfusion ratios, due to the anatomical alterations found in COPD, is the predominant mechanism accounting for abnormal gas exchange. Reduced ventilation may be due to reduced ventilatory drive and the high work of breathing because of severe airflow limitation and hyperinflation plus ventilatory muscle impairment which may lead to carbon dioxide retention. The extent of impairment of diffusing capacity for carbon monoxide is the best physiological correlate to the severity of emphysema.

### Pulmonary hypertension

Pulmonary hypertension develops late in the course of COPD at the time of severe gas exchange abnormalities, and is initially due to hypoxic pulmonary arterial vasoconstriction. An inflammatory response in vessels occurs similar to that found within airways along with endothelial cell dysfunction. This can lead to structural changes that include intimal hyperplasia and smooth muscle hypertrophy/hyperplasia and destruction of the pulmonary capillary bed. The development of structural changes in the pulmonary arterioles results in persistent pulmonary hypertension and right ventricular hypertrophy/enlargement and dysfunction (Figure 2.5).

### Systemic effects

COPD is associated with several extrapulmonary effects (Box 2.5). The systemic inflammation and skeletal muscle wasting contribute to exercise capacity limitation and worsen prognosis, irrespective of the degree of airflow obstruction. There is an increased risk of cardiovascular disease in individuals with COPD and, if present, it is associated with a systemic inflammatory response and vascular dysfunction.

Box 2.5 **Systemic features of COPD.**

- Cachexia
- Skeletal muscle wasting
- Increased risk of cardiovascular disease
- Normochromic normocytic anaemia
- Osteoporosis
- Depression
- Secondary polycythaemia

## Pathology, pathogenesis and pathophysiology of exacerbations

Exacerbations are often associated with increased neutrophilic inflammation in the airways and in others, increased numbers of eosinophils are found. Some exacerbations are infectious in origin (either bacterial or viral), while other potential mechanisms include air pollution and changes in ambient temperature. Viruses and bacteria may activate transcription factors such as NF-κB and the MAP kinases, leading to the release of inflammatory cytokines.

In mild exacerbations, the degree of airflow limitation is often unchanged or only slightly increased. Severe exacerbations are associated with worsening of pulmonary gas exchange due to increased ventilation/perfusion inequality and subsequent respiratory muscle fatigue. The worsening ventilation/perfusion relationship is due to airway inflammation, oedema, mucous hypersecretion and bronchoconstriction. These reduce ventilation and cause hypoxic vasoconstriction of pulmonary arterioles, which in turn impairs perfusion.

Respiratory muscle fatigue and alveolar hypoventilation can contribute to hypoxaemia, hypercapnia, respiratory acidosis and lead to severe respiratory failure and death. Hypoxia and respiratory acidosis can induce pulmonary vasoconstriction, which increases the load on the right ventricle and, together with renal hormonal changes, can result in peripheral oedema (cor pulmonale).

## Further reading

Bagdonas E, Raudoniute J, Bruzauskaite L, Aldonyte R. Novel aspects of pathogenesis and regeneration mechanisms in COPD. *International Journal of COPD* 2015; **10**: 995–1013.

Barnes PJ. Cellular and molecular mechanisms of chronic obstructive pulmonary disease. *Clinics in Chest Medicine* 2014; **35**: 71–86.

Caramori G, Kirkham P, Barczyk A, di Stefano A, Adcock I. Molecular pathogenesis of cigarette smoking-induced stable COPD. *Annals of the New York Academy of Sciences* 2015; **1340**: 55–64.

Hogg JC, Timens W. The pathology of chronic obstructive pulmonary disease. *Annual Review of Pathology* 2009; **4**: 435–459.

# CHAPTER 3

# Diagnosis

*Graeme P. Currie, David R. Miller and Mahendran Chetty*

Aberdeen Royal Infirmary, Aberdeen, UK

---

**OVERVIEW**

- Consider chronic obstructive pulmonary disease (COPD) in individuals >35 years with breathlessness, chest tightness, wheeze, cough, sputum production, frequent chest infections and reduced exercise tolerance with a history of smoking (or other significant risk factor).

- Recording the COPD assessment test (CAT) or modified Medical Research Council (mMRC) scores helps quantify the impact of COPD on overall health and well-being, and guide therapy.

- Clinical examination may be normal, especially in early disease.

- Perform spirometry in all patients with suspected COPD to confirm the diagnosis and grade the severity of airflow obstruction.

- Perform a chest X-ray and full blood count at the time of diagnosis to help exclude other causes of breathlessness.

- Consider other investigations such as detailed lung function tests, electrocardiogram, echocardiogram, chest computed tomography and arterial blood gases, depending on the clinical circumstances.

---

As with most medical conditions, take a thorough history and perform a clinical examination before embarking on investigations in a patient with possible or suspected COPD. Consider the diagnosis in individuals over 35 years of age with any relevant respiratory symptom and history of smoking or other significant risk factor (e.g. passive smoking or exposure to indoor biomass fuels in developing countries). The presence of airflow obstruction and its severity are confirmed by postbronchodilator spirometry; this remains the gold standard diagnostic test (see Chapter 4).

## Clinical features

### Typical presenting symptoms

COPD may be present in any current or former smoker over the age of 35 years who complains of breathlessness, chest tightness, wheeze, chronic cough, sputum production, frequent winter chest infections or impaired exercise tolerance. Symptoms such as breathlessness, chest tightness and wheeze which occur primarily overnight are more suggestive of asthma, while breathlessness alone overnight may reflect paroxysmal nocturnal dyspnoea. COPD may be present in the absence of troublesome respiratory symptoms, especially in those with a sedentary lifestyle or limited mobility.

Breathlessness (an undue awareness of breathing) is a symptom perceived by the patient (and not a clinical sign); some patients may describe it as 'shortness of breath' or 'difficulty getting enough air in'. It may only initially be perceived during marked exertion, although it typically becomes progressive and persistent. In COPD, the development of breathlessness is generally insidious over months or years. It is useful to determine how breathlessness effects daily living activities such as walking on the flat (and walking distance), walking up inclines, climbing flights of stairs, carrying bags, walking to the shops, washing and dressing, performing light housework, work and hobbies; some patients with advanced COPD complain of difficulty in eating and talking due to breathlessness. The impact of breathlessness on an individual's day-to-day life can be objectively assessed by the modified Medical Research Council (mMRC) dyspnoea scale (Table 3.1).

Chest tightness and wheeze (the high-pitched noise produced by air travelling through abnormally narrowed smaller airways) can occur at rest and exertion, but may only be experienced upon exertion or during an exacerbation.

Cough is a forced expulsive manoevre against an initially closed glottis. Chronic cough (defined as lasting >8 weeks) may be the presenting symptom in many other respiratory disorders (Table 3.2). In COPD, it is usually associated with sputum production. In healthy individuals, around 100 mL of sputum is produced daily, which is transported up the airway and swallowed; expectoration of excessive amounts of sputum is usually abnormal. In COPD, excessive amounts of sputum are often expectorated in the mornings and tends to be clear (mucoid), although it may also be light green because of overnight stagnation of neutrophils and other inflammatory cells. During an exacerbation, sputum is usually greater in quantity than usual and may be dark green because of dead neutrophils. Particularly large volumes of purulent (pus-containing) sputum production, typically on a regular basis, occurs in bronchiectasis.

---

*ABC of COPD*, Third Edition. Edited by Graeme P. Currie.

**Table 3.1** Modified Medical Research Council breathlessness scale.

| Grade | Degree of breathlessness related to activities |
|-------|------------------------------------------------|
| 0 | I only get breathless with strenuous exercise |
| 1 | I get short of breath when hurrying on the level or walking up a slight hill |
| 2 | I walk slower than people of the same age on the level because of breathlessness, or I have to stop for breath when walking at my own pace on the level |
| 3 | I stop for breath after walking about 100 metres or after a few minutes on the level |
| 4 | I am too breathless to leave the house or I am breathless when dressing or undressing |

**Table 3.2** Causes of a chronic (lasting >8 weeks) cough.

| Airway disorders | Parenchymal diseases | Pleural diseases | Other conditions |
|------------------|---------------------|------------------|------------------|
| COPD | Lung cancer | Pleural effusion | Gastro-oesophageal reflux disease |
| Asthma | Idiopathic pulmonary fibrosis | Mesothelioma | Upper airway cough syndrome |
| Bronchiectasis | Chronic lung infections (TB or fungal infections) | | Angiotensin-converting enzyme inhibitor use |
| Smoker's cough/chronic bronchitis | Extrinsic allergic alveolitis | | Exposure to irritant dusts/chemicals/fumes/particulate matter |
| Eosinophilic bronchitis | | | |
| Postviral hyperreactivity | | | |

COPD, chronic obstructive pulmonary disease; TB, tuberculosis.

## Other features in the history

The initial presenting feature of COPD may be with repeated lower respiratory tract infections, especially during winter months. Haemoptysis is not a feature of COPD and its presence should always raise the suspicion of a serious underlying disorder such as lung cancer or other conditions such as pulmonary embolism, pulmonary oedema, an underlying vasculitis (granulomatosis with polyangiitis or Goodpasture syndrome) or infection (e.g. tuberculosis, lung abscess, bronchiectasis or occasionally pneumonia).

As part of the overall assessment of COPD, find out about:
- previous chest problems (e.g. asthma or tuberculosis)
- other medical conditions (such as cardiovascular disease, diabetes, osteoporosis, depression and anxiety)
- frequency of exacerbations (and number of courses of steroids and antibiotics in the preceding year)
- number of hospital admissions
- exercise limitation
- number of days missed from work
- current medication and inhalers (doses, frequency and adherence)
- financial impact and the extent of social and family support.

Ask also about occupational and environmental exposure to dust, chemicals and fumes, biomass fuel (especially in less well developed countries), and pets; in particular, ask about contact with birds (such as pigeons, parrots and parakeets) as some patients may have concomitant extrinsic allergic alveolitis. Enquire if patients have been exposed to asbestos; occupations at particular risk of exposure include welders, joiners, marine engineers and shipyard workers. Such individuals may have pleural plaques and pleural thickening (which, in isolation, do not usually cause symptoms) and are at a heightened risk of developing lung cancer (especially if there is a history of cigarette smoking), asbestosis, benign or malignant pleural effusions or malignant pleural mesothelioma.

There is increasing evidence that COPD causes systemic effects, with loss of skeletal muscle mass, anorexia and weight loss being relatively common and underrecognised problems. Recent weight gain may also compound symptoms of COPD which in itself may be the sole explanation behind an apparent deterioration.

## Assessing the impact of COPD

The overall measure of health status impairment (i.e. quality of life) can be determined objectively by various assessment questionnaires, for example the St George's Respiratory Questionnaire (SGRQ) and COPD Assessment Test (CAT). The SGRQ is validated, reliable and repeatable, and assesses three main domains: symptoms, activity and psychosocial impact. It takes up to 15 minutes to complete, and is often used in clinical trials before, during and after an intervention to determine presence and extent of any responses. A reduction in score of 4 units in the SGRQ is considered to be clinically relevant.

The CAT is a validated 8-item, more simple questionnaire (which takes only a couple of minutes for the patient to complete) with scoring range of 0–40 (Box 3.1). It helps patients and clinicians determine the overall impact of COPD and provides complementary information to measurements of lung function and frequency of exacerbations. Values (and changes in values) recorded by the CAT can occur with changes in COPD and treatment. Based on a minimally clinically important difference of 4 in the SGRQ, a change of at least 2 in the CAT is considered to be broadly comparable. International guidelines advocate that the CAT (and/or mMRC) score is determined to categorise patients into groups A, B, C or D as a guide to optimise management.

## Smoking history

Determine when a patient started smoking, when he/she stopped smoking, the number of cigarettes smoked each day, current smoking status and use of e-cigarettes (with or without traditional cigarettes). Ask patients about willingness to quit smoking and consider referral to smoking cessation services. The number of smoking pack-years can be calculated as follows.
- One pack-year is defined as 20 cigarettes (one pack) smoked per day for 1 year.
- Number of pack years = (number of cigarettes smoked per day × number of years smoked)/20.
- For example, a patient who has smoked 15 cigarettes per day for 40 years has a $(15 \times 40)/20 = 30$ pack-year smoking history.

Box 3.1 **The COPD Assessment Test. Reproduced with permission from GlaxoSmithKline.**

| Your name: | | Today's date: | | **CAT**™ |
| --- | --- | --- | --- | --- |
| | | | | COPD Assessment Test |

# How is your COPD? Take the COPD Assessment Test™ (CAT)

This questionnaire will help you and your healthcare professional measure the impact COPD (Chronic Obstructive Pulmonary Disease) is having on your wellbeing and daily life. Your answers, and test score, can be used by you and your healthcare professional to help improve the management of your COPD and get the greatest benefit from treatment.

For each item below, place a mark (X) in the box that best describes you currently. Be sure to only select one response for each question.

**Example:** I am very happy ⓪ Ⓧ ② ③ ④ ⑤ I am very sad

SCORE

| I never cough | ⓪ ① ② ③ ④ ⑤ | I cough all the time | |
| --- | --- | --- | --- |
| I have no phlegm (mucus) in my chest at all | ⓪ ① ② ③ ④ ⑤ | My chest is completely full of phlegm (mucus) | |
| My chest does not feel tight at all | ⓪ ① ② ③ ④ ⑤ | My chest feels very tight | |
| When I walk up a hill or one flight of stairs I am not breathless | ⓪ ① ② ③ ④ ⑤ | When I walk up a hill or one flight of stairs I am very breathless | |
| I am not limited doing any activities at home | ⓪ ① ② ③ ④ ⑤ | I am very limited doing activities at home | |
| I am confident leaving my home despite my lung condition | ⓪ ① ② ③ ④ ⑤ | I am not at all confident leaving my home because of my lung condition | |
| I sleep soundly | ⓪ ① ② ③ ④ ⑤ | I don't sleep soundly because of my lung condition | |
| I have lots of energy | ⓪ ① ② ③ ④ ⑤ | I have no energy at all | |

**TOTAL SCORE**

## Signs

Signs of respiratory disease tend to appear as COPD progresses. Physical examination may therefore be normal, or alternatively reveal only prolongation of the expiratory phase of respiration or an elevated respiratory rate (tachypnoea) at rest in mild disease (the normal resting respiratory rate in healthy adults is 12–18 breaths per minute). In COPD, wheeze is usually heard during expiration (as airways normally dilate during inspiration and narrow during expiration) and may occur only during exercise, in the morning (reflecting pooling of secretions blocking off smaller airways) or during an exacerbation. Late course inspiratory crackles are occasionally found in COPD, especially when excessive lower airway secretions are present.

As the disease progresses, examination may reveal a hyperinflated chest, increased anteroposterior diameter of the chest wall, intercostal indrawing, diminished breath sounds, wheezing at rest and faint heart sounds (due to hyperinflated lungs). Cyanosis (blue discolouration of the skin, lips and mucous membranes (Figure 3.1)), pursed lip breathing and use of accessory muscles (sternocleidomastoids, platysma and pectoral muscles) are features of advanced disease.

Stridor (a harsh croaking noise on inspiration) and hoarseness are not found in COPD and other conditions (such as large airway obstruction and laryngeal nerve palsy respectively) should be considered; hoarseness is, however, a common adverse effect of moderate to high doses of inhaled corticosteroids.

Cor pulmonale is present when right ventricular hypertrophy and pulmonary hypertension occur as a consequence of any chronic lung disorder. Some patients with advanced COPD may therefore demonstrate signs consistent with cor pulmonale (raised jugular venous pressure, loud P2 due to pulmonary hypertension, tricuspid regurgitation, pitting peripheral oedema (Figure 3.2) and hepatomegaly) and its presence usually indicates a poor prognosis. It may occur alongside features of $CO_2$ retention (warm peripheries, peripheral vasodilation and bounding pulse). Finger clubbing is *not* found in COPD and its presence should prompt thorough evaluation to exclude a cause such as lung cancer, bronchiectasis or idiopathic pulmonary fibrosis (Figure 3.3). Tar staining of the nails and fingers is commonly found in current or previous heavy cigarette smokers with COPD (Figure 3.4).

Skeletal muscle wasting and cachexia may occur in advanced disease, while some patients may also be overweight. The body mass index (BMI; weight (kg)/height (m)$^2$) is a measure for calculating the nutritional status of adults; determine this during the initial examination (Table 3.3).

The BODE index (BMI, Obstruction, Dyspnoea and Exercise) is a grading system which predicts the risk of death from any cause and from respiratory causes among patients with COPD (Table 3.4). A BODE index of 0–2, 3–4, 5–6 and 7–10 is thought to

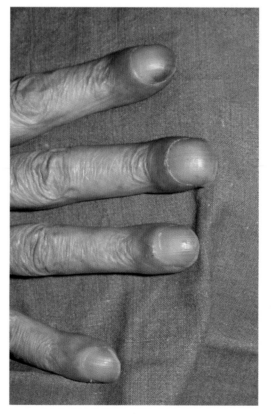

**Figure 3.2** Pitting ankle oedema is a feature of cor pulmonale; consider other causes or contributory factors such as oral corticosteroids, calcium channel antagonists, excessive intravenous fluid administration, hypoalbumenaemia or dependant oedema.

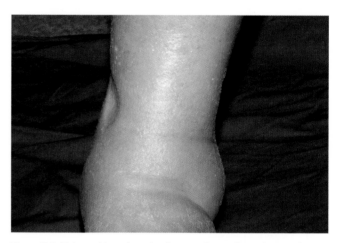

**Figure 3.3** A patient with tar staining and finger clubbing; chronic obstructive pulmonary disease and non-small cell lung cancer were both diagnosed in this patient.

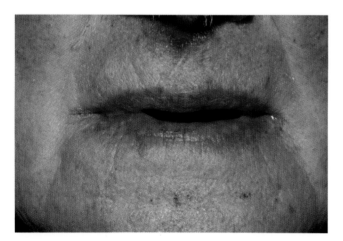

**Figure 3.1** A patient with advanced hypoxic chronic obstructive pulmonary disease with central cyanosis.

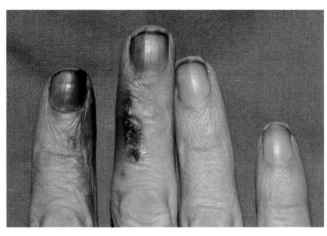

**Figure 3.4** A right-handed patient with gross tar staining of the fingers due to chronic cigarette smoking.

**Table 3.3** World Health Organization classification of body mass index (BMI) and nutritional status.

| BMI | Nutritional status |
|---|---|
| <18.5 | Underweight |
| 18.5–24.9 | Normal weight |
| 25.0–29.9 | Pre-obesity |
| 30.0–34.9 | Obesity class I |
| 35.0–39.9 | Obesity class II |
| ≥40 | Obesity class III |

**Table 3.4** Calculation of the BODE index.

| Parameter | Points | | | | |
|---|---|---|---|---|---|
| | 0 | 1 | 2 | 3 | Score |
| BMI | ≤21 | >21 | | | 0 or 1 |
| FEV₁ % predicted | ≥65 | 50–64 | 36–49 | ≤35 | 0, 1, 2 or 3 |
| Modified MRC scale | 0–1 | 2 | 3 | 4 | 0, 1, 2 or 3 |
| 6-minute walk distance (metres) | ≥350 | 250–349 | 150–249 | ≤149 | 0, 1, 2 or 3 |
| | | | | | Total (out of 10) |

The modified MRC scale uses the same clinical descriptors as the original MRC scale (1–5), although respective values are denoted as 0–4 in the calculation of the BODE index.
BODE, BMI, Obstruction, Dyspnoea and Exercise; FEV$_1$, forced expiratory volume in 1 second; MRC, Medical Research Council.

be associated with a 52-month mortality rate of approximately 10%, 30%, 50% and 80% respectively.

## Differential diagnosis

Pay particular attention to other features in the history and examination, which may indicate an alternative or concomitant disorder (Table 3.5). Since asthma tends to be the main differential diagnosis of COPD, take a detailed history in order to help distinguish between either disorder (Table 3.6). So-called 'red flag' symptoms such as haemoptysis, chest pain and weight loss usually require urgent referral to secondary care to rule out lung cancer or an alternative cardiorespiratory disorder.

## Investigations

### Lung function testing

Solitary peak expiratory flow (PEF) readings can significantly and seriously underestimate the extent of airflow obstruction, while serial monitoring of PEF is not generally useful in the diagnosis of COPD. Demonstration of airflow obstruction with spirometry is required to confirm the diagnosis. Postbronchodilator spirometry is also useful in assessing severity of the disease and in following its progress plus response to treatment. The normal age-related decline in forced expiratory volume in 1 second (FEV$_1$) is approximately 20–40 mL/year and this increases to approximately 40–80 mL/year in current smokers. More detailed lung function measurements such as lung volumes (total lung capacity and residual volume), gas transfer and 6-minute walk test can be performed if doubt exists in diagnosis or more thorough evaluation is required (such as during assessment for surgery or lung transplantation). Lung function testing in COPD is discussed in detail in Chapter 4 (Figure 3.5).

### Imaging

All patients with suspected COPD should have a posteroanterior chest X-ray performed at diagnosis (Figure 3.6). This may be normal although as the disease progresses, features of hyperinflation (flattened diaphragms, a narrowed heart, >6 anterior rib ends visible and 'squared-off apices') and hyperlucency of lung fields may be evident. A chest X-ray also helps discount other causes of respiratory symptoms and identify complications related to COPD such as bullae formation and pulmonary arterial hypertension (enlarged central pulmonary arteries and peripheral arterial pruning). There is no direct link between extent of chest X-ray abnormality and

**Table 3.5** Conditions in the differential diagnosis of COPD.

| Condition | Suggestive feature | Investigation |
|---|---|---|
| Asthma | Family history, presence of other atopic disorders, non-smoker, young age, nocturnal symptoms | Trial of inhaled corticosteroids, reversibility testing if airflow obstruction present |
| Congestive cardiac failure | Orthopnoea, history of ischaemic heart disease, fine lung crackles, atrial fibrillation, hypertension | Chest X-ray, electrocardiogram, echocardiogram |
| Lung cancer | Haemoptysis, weight loss, hoarseness, extensive smoking history | Chest X-ray, bronchoscopy, CT |
| Bronchiectasis | Daily purulent sputum production, frequent chest infections, childhood pneumonia, coarse lung crackles | Sputum microscopy, culture and sensitivity, high-resolution CT |
| Interstitial lung disease | Dry cough, history of connective tissue disease, use of drugs such as methotrexate, amiodarone, nitrofurantoin, etc., fine lung crackles | Pulmonary function testing, chest X-ray, high-resolution CT, lung biopsy, autoantibodies |
| Opportunistic infection | Dry cough, risk factors for immunosuppression, fever | Chest X-ray, sputum microscopy, culture and sensitivity, induced sputum, bronchoalveolar lavage |
| Tuberculosis | Weight loss, haemoptysis, night sweats, risk factors for tuberculosis and immunosuppression | Chest X-ray, sputum microscopy, culture and sensitivity |

COPD, chronic obstructive pulmonary disease; CT, computed tomography.

**Table 3.6** Clinical differences between COPD and asthma.

|  | COPD | Asthma |
|---|---|---|
| Age | >35 years | Any age |
| Cough | Persistent and productive | Intermittent and non-productive |
| Smoking | Almost invariable | Possible |
| Breathlessness | Progressive and persistent | Intermittent and variable |
| Nocturnal symptoms | Uncommon unless in severe disease | Common |
| Family history | Uncommon unless family members also smoke | Common |
| Concomitant eczema or allergic rhinitis | Possible | Common |

COPD, chronic obstructive pulmonary disease.

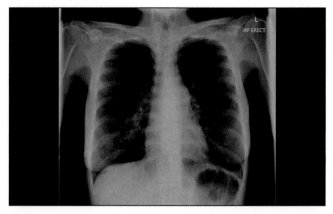

**Figure 3.6** Chest radiograph showing typical changes of advanced COPD (>6 ends of anterior rib visible, flat diaphragms, increased translucency of lung fields and 'squared-off' lung apices).

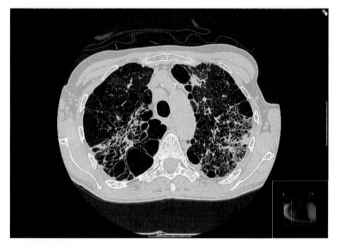

**Figure 3.7** High-resolution computed tomogram of the chest showing widespread upper lobe emphysematous bullae in a patient with advanced COPD.

**Table 3.7** Secondary polycythaemia in a male with advanced hypoxic chronic obstructive pulmonary disease. Typically, blood parameters demonstrate an increase in haemoglobin concentration accompanied by an elevated red cell count and haematocrit. This patient had an elevated white cell count (neutrophilia) due to high-dose oral corticosteroids.

| Parameter | Actual result | Typical normal range |
|---|---|---|
| Haemoglobin | 178 g/L | 116–156 g/L |
| Red cell count | $6.1 \times 10^{12}$/L | $3.8–5.2 \times 10^{12}$/L |
| Mean corpuscular volume | 84 fl | 83–98 fl |
| Haematocrit | 0.54 L/L | 0.34–0.51 L/L |
| Platelet count | $200 \times 10^9$/L | $140–400 \times 10^9$/L |
| White cell count | $15.2 \times 10^9$/L | $4.0–10.0 \times 10^9$/L |

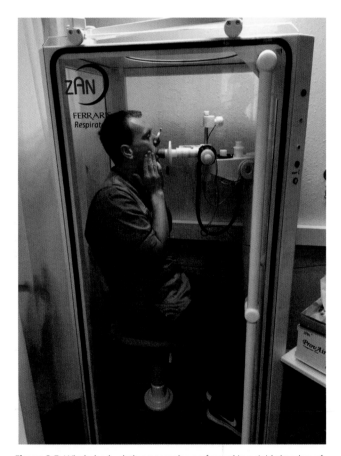

**Figure 3.5** Whole-body plethysmography, performed in a rigid chamber of comparable size and shape to a telephone booth, can be used to measure lung volumes.

degree of airflow obstruction. When there is doubt in diagnosis or an interventional procedure is contemplated (such as endoscopic lung volume reduction, lung volume reduction surgery or bullectomy), high-resolution computed tomographic (HRCT) imaging of the chest is required (Figure 3.7).

## Other investigations

Check a full blood count in all patients at the time of diagnosis; this may show secondary polycythaemia, and excludes anaemia as a cause of chronic breathlessness (Table 3.7). The discovery of a raised eosinophil count should suggest the possibility of an alternative diagnosis such as asthma or eosinophilic pneumonia.

In patients with signs of cor pulmonale, an electrocardiogram may show changes of chronic right-sided heart strain (Figure 3.8). However, an echocardiogram is more sensitive in detecting tricuspid valve incompetence along with right atrial and ventricular hypertrophy and may also indirectly assess pulmonary artery pressure. Moreover, echocardiography is also a useful tool to determine

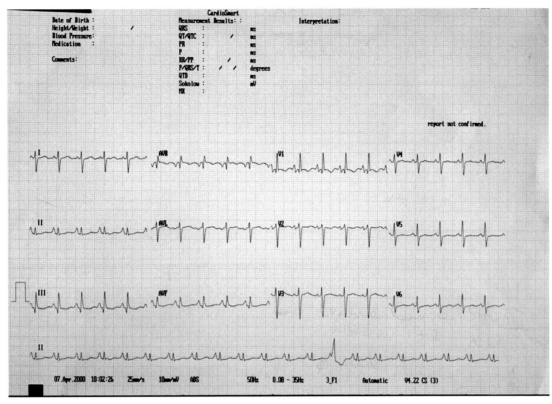

**Figure 3.8** Electrocardiogram showing typical changes in a patient with cor pulmonale (p-pulmonale, right axis deviation, partial right bundle branch block).

whether left ventricular dysfunction is present, especially when the spirometric impairment is disproportionate to the extent of breathlessness. It is also important to be aware that ischaemic heart disease may be the sole or contributory cause of breathlessness (anginal equivalent), even in the absence of chest pain, and investigations should be tailored accordingly. Indeed, dyspnoea due to causes other than COPD should be considered when the extent of physical limitation appears disproportionate to the degree of airflow obstruction.

α1-Antitrypsin deficiency is an autosomal co-dominant genetic disorder associated with the early development of airflow obstruction, panacinar emphysema and liver dysfunction. Necrotising panniculitis and granulomatosis with polyangiitis (previously known as Wegener's granulomatosis) are infrequent complications. Individuals with a family history of COPD, or when it presents at a young age (especially when smoking pack-years are negligible), should have α1-antitrypsin levels checked. If α1-antitrypsin deficiency is discovered, family screening and counselling, along with strict advice on smoking cessation, are warranted.

Assessment of pulse oximetry is useful in most patients, especially when more advanced disease ($FEV_1 < 50\%$ predicted) or secondary polycythaemia polycythaemia is present, to detect the possibility of significant hypoxaemia. Patients with a resting oxygen saturation of <92% should have measurement of arterial blood gases, and where necessary and appropriate, be considered for assessment for long-term domiciliary or ambulatory oxygen.

## Further reading

Celli BR, Cote CG, Marin JM et al. The body-mass index, airflow obstruction, dyspnea, and exercise capacity index in chronic obstructive pulmonary disease. *New England Journal of Medicine* 2004; **350**: 1005–1012.

http://guidance.nice.org.uk/CG101/Guidance/pdf/English

Jones PW, Quirk FH, Baveystock CM, Littlejohns P. A self-complete measure for chronic airflow limitation – the St George's Respiratory Questionnaire. *American Review of Respiratory Disease* 1992; **145**: 1321–1327.

http://catestonline.org

Vogelmeier CF, Criner GJ, Martinez FJ, et al. Global Strategy for the Diagnosis, Management, and Prevention of Chronic Obstructive Lung Disease 2017 Report. *Eur Respir J* 2017; **49**: 1700214 [https://doi.org/10.1183/13993003.00214-2017].

# CHAPTER 4

# Spirometry

*Claire Fotheringham*

Aberdeen Royal Infirmary, Aberdeen, UK

---

**OVERVIEW**

- Spirometry is an essential investigation in the diagnosis (and exclusion) of chronic obstructive pulmonary disease (COPD) and in quantifying the degree of airflow obstruction.
- When consistent symptoms are present, clinically significant COPD can usually be diagnosed when forced expiratory volume in 1 second/forced vital capacity ($FEV_1$/FVC) <0.7 *and* $FEV_1$ <80% predicted.
- Along with assessment of clinical features, spirometry can help differentiate COPD from asthma and other respiratory disorders.
- Spirometry curves and values – when performed correctly on calibrated, well-maintained spirometers – are accurate, reliable and repeatable.
- Approved educational courses for operators – or at the very least comprehensive and supervised training by an experienced and competent mentor certified in performing spirometry – are essential in the provision of a high-quality, worthwhile service.

---

## Introduction

While history and examination are essential in the diagnostic work-up of suspected chronic obstructive pulmonary disease (COPD), demonstrating airflow obstruction is vital in confirming (or refuting) the diagnosis. Spirometry is recommended as being mandatory by all national guidelines and should therefore be arranged for all individuals in whom the diagnosis of COPD is considered. Without incorporating spirometry routinely into a respiratory service, whether in primary or secondary care, patients may receive an inaccurate diagnosis and the disease severity can be incorrectly estimated.

Spirometry was traditionally only performed in hospital lung function laboratories and respiratory outpatient clinics. In recent years, there has been a major shift in accessibility with it now being routinely performed in primary care settings. However, major concerns regarding technical performance, quality and interpretation of results in primary care have been raised and it

has been acknowledged that training for members of the primary care team can be highly variable and inconsistent. This all implies a need for attendance at accredited courses.

## What is spirometry?

Spirometry is a method of assessing lung function by measuring the volume of air that can be expelled from the lungs following maximal inspiration. Values derived from this forced expiratory manoeuvre have become the most accurate, repeatable and reliable way of helping confirm or refute the presence of airflow obstruction. Absolute values obtained from an individual can be compared to their predicted values.

## Why perform spirometry?

Spirometry is the best way of detecting the presence of airflow obstruction and helping to establish a definitive diagnosis of COPD. To make a diagnosis of clinically significant COPD, the postbronchodilator forced expiratory volume in 1 second ($FEV_1$)/forced vital capacity (FVC) ratio, or FEVR, needs to be less than 0.7 *and* $FEV_1$ below 80% predicted. If $FEV_1$ is ≥80% predicted of normal, a diagnosis of COPD should only be made at the discretion of a clinician.

Repeating spirometry over a period of time can be useful for assessing response to treatment and monitoring and quantifying disease progression. Demonstration of abnormal lung function may even help motivate individuals who smoke to quit. Consider an alternative diagnosis in older patients without typical symptoms of COPD even if the FEVR is <0.7 and in younger patients with symptoms of COPD where the FEVR is ≥0.7. This is due to age-related differences in expected lung function values.

## Types of spirometer

Different types of spirometers exist and are used in various clinical settings. Large wedge bellows or rolling-seal spirometers are not portable and are used mainly in lung function laboratories. They

---

*ABC of COPD*, Third Edition. Edited by Graeme P. Currie.

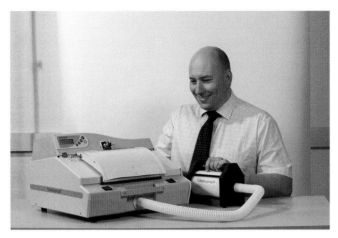

**Figure 4.1** A wedge bellows spirometer being calibrated.

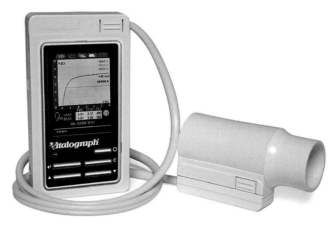

**Figure 4.3** A hand-held spirometer.

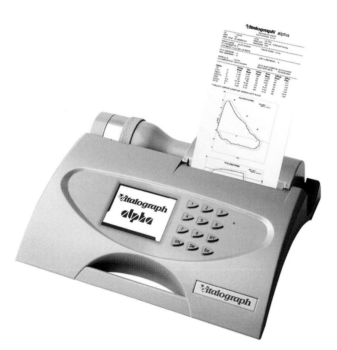

**Figure 4.2** A desktop spirometer.

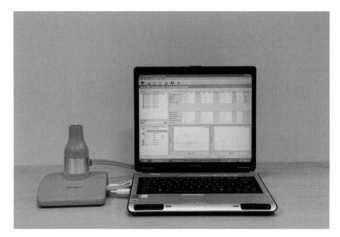

**Figure 4.4** Some hand-held spirometers can deliver results directly to computers.

are useful for screening in primary and secondary care, and providing they can be either calibrated or verified prior to use, allow for an accurate diagnosis.

Many spirometers provide two types of traces:
- volume of air exhaled versus time
- flow versus volume of air exhaled (or flow/volume curve).

## How to perform spirometry

Perform spirometry when the patient is clinically stable and feeling well. Ideally, withhold short-acting bronchodilators for at least the previous 4 hours, long-acting bronchodilators for atleast 24 hours and sustained-release theophylline, inhaled corticosteroids and combination inhalers containing long-acting bronchodilators (long-acting $\beta_2$-agonists and/or long-acting muscarinic antagonists) for atleast 24 hours prior to performing the test. When performing spirometry for the first time, most patients, once comfortably seated, need clear, concise and unhurried instruction by a skilled and experienced operator (Box 4.1).

require regular calibration but provide very accurate measurements (Figure 4.1). Desktop spirometers are compact, portable and quick and easy to use (Figure 4.2). They usually have a real-time visual display and often provide a paper printout. Some types require calibration and others can have their accuracy verified with a 3 L syringe; in the case of the latter, changes need to be made by the manufacturer. Generally, desktop spirometers require little maintenance other than cleaning and regular servicing, and are ideal for use in primary care by an appropriately trained operator. Smaller inexpensive hand-held spirometers provide a numerical record of forced expiratory manoeuvre values; a printout of results from this type of device is not always possible (Figures 4.3, 4.4). Spirometers

**Table 4.1** Causes of obstructive and restrictive spirometry.

| Obstructive disorders | Restrictive disorders |
|---|---|
| Chronic obstructive pulmonary disease | Neuromuscular disorders |
| Symptomatic asthma | Interstitial lung disease |
| Bronchiectasis | Kyphoscoliosis |
| | Large pleural effusion |
| | Morbid obesity |
| | Previous pneumonectomy |

**Table 4.2** Typical features of normal, obstructive, restrictive and mixed obstructive/restrictive spirometry.

| Pattern | $FEV_1$ | FVC | FEVR ($FEV_1$/FVC) |
|---|---|---|---|
| Normal | ≥80% predicted | ≥80% predicted | 0.7–0.8 |
| Obstructive | <80% predicted | >80% predicted (or <80% predicted in advanced disease) | <0.7 |
| Restrictive | <80% predicted | <80% predicted ($FEV_1$ and FVC reduced proportionately) | ≥0.85 (although often ≥0.7) |
| Mixed obstructive/ restrictive | <80% predicted | <80% predicted ($FEV_1$ reduced to a greater extent than FVC) | <0.7 |

$FEV_1$, forced expiratory volume in 1 second; FEVR, forced expiratory volume in 1 second ($FEV_1$)/forced vital capacity (FVC) ratio; FVC, forced vital capacity.

## Spirometric indices

The standard manoeuvre is a maximal forced exhalation (with greatest effort possible) after a maximum deep inspiration (from total lung capacity). Several indices can be derived from this manoeuvre:

- FVC – the total volume of air that can be forcibly exhaled in one breath
- $FEV_1$ – the volume of air that can be exhaled in the first second of forced expiration
- FEVR or $FEV_1$/FVC – the ratio of $FEV_1$ to FVC (expressed as a decimal).

The $FEV_1$ and FVC are measured in litres and also expressed as a percentage of the predicted value for the individual. Predicted values are derived from 'normal' individuals and vary with gender, height, age and ethnicity. The most up-to-date predicted values are those published by the Global Lung Initiative in 2012. These updated equations are more age and ethnic origin appropriate for use globally than European Community Health and Respiratory Survey equations previously recommended for European populations. Operators should be aware of the predicted equations selected for use by their equipment and ensure that the equation most appropriate for the local population is used. Depending on the year of manufacture, Global Lung Initiative 2012 equations may not be available for selection. This should be a key consideration when purchasing a spirometer.

The FEVR is normally between 0.7 and 0.8. Values <0.7 indicate airflow obstruction, although in older adults, values between 0.65 and 0.7 may be normal. Using 0.7 as a cut-off may therefore lead to overdiagnosis of COPD in the elderly, meaning that age should be taken into consideration when making a diagnosis. The FEVR is expected to be ≥0.85 in restrictive ventilatory defects (although often ≥0.7). Typical causes of obstructive and restrictive ventilatory defects are shown in Table 4.1. Key features of spirometric indices found in individuals with normal spirometry and different types of ventilatory defects are summarised in Table 4.2.

## Other measurements

### Forced expiratory volume in 6 seconds ($FEV_6$)

This is a more recently derived value, which measures the volume of air that can be forcibly exhaled in 6 seconds. It approximates the FVC, and in healthy individuals, the $FEV_6$ and FVC are identical. Using $FEV_6$ instead of FVC may be helpful in patients with more severe airflow obstruction as a quantifiable measurement when no plateau in exhaled volume can be achieved.

### Slow vital capacity (SVC) (also known as relaxed VC (RVC) or VC)

This parameter is obtained when the patient inhales to total lung capacity and performs a controlled, steady maximal exhalation. In patients with more advanced airflow obstruction and dynamic compression, the slow VC may exceed the FVC and is a useful parameter to measure, usually prior to performing FVC.

### Inspired vital capacity (IVC)

This measurement of vital capacity is the maximal volume that can be inhaled from the point of maximal exhalation. International guidelines suggest that IVC or SVC can be used instead of FVC in the FEVR if a higher value is obtained in those measurements.

### Forced midexpiratory flow (FEF$_{25-75}$)

This is the flow of air forcibly exhaled between 25% and 75% of the FVC manoeuvre; it is often thought to be reflective of airflow obstruction in smaller airways.

## Interpretation and classification of spirograms

Interpretation of spirometry involves evaluating absolute values of FEV$_1$, FVC and FEVR, comparing them with predicted values and examining the shape of traces. Patients should complete three acceptable manoeuvres which have the two best FVC and FEV$_1$ values within 5% or 100 mL of each other; some electronic spirometers automatically provide this information. Record the best FVC and FEV$_1$, although they do not need to be taken from the same effort.

Flow/volume interpretation is a helpful addition to understanding results and provides a quick and simple check as to whether airflow obstruction is present. It may also identify early stages of airflow obstruction and provide additional information when interpreting a mixed pattern of obstruction and restriction.

Examples of spirometric traces (volume/time shown above and flow/volume shown below) in different respiratory classifications are shown in Figure 4.5. The red line represents the normal curve and the blue line represents a patient with an abnormal curve.

## Bronchodilator reversibility testing

In most patients, reversibility testing is not necessary since asthma can usually be differentiated from COPD on clinical features and baseline spirometry. It is important to remember that response to treatment is not predicted by acute reversibility testing. Clinically significant COPD is not present if the FEV$_1$ and FEVR return to normal with treatment (bronchodilator and/or steroids).

To help resolve cases where diagnostic doubt remains, or when both COPD and asthma may be present, the following features are highly suggestive of asthma:
- >400 mL improvement in FEV$_1$ following inhaled bronchodilators
- >400 mL improvement in FEV$_1$ following 30 mg oral prednisolone daily for 2 weeks.

Other authorities indicate that a 'positive' response to inhaled bronchodilator is suggested by a 12% improvement in FEV$_1$ and 200 mL improvement in FEV$_1$ or FVC.

## Severity of airflow obstruction in COPD

The severity of airflow obstruction in COPD can be categorised according to the degree of impairment of FEV$_1$% predicted (Table 4.3).

## Accuracy and quality of traces

Examples of poor technique for varying reasons are shown in Figure 4.6. The most common cause for poor-quality spirometry is suboptimal patient effort (sometimes due to inadequate, hurried or poor explanation by the operator). It is therefore important to observe the patient throughout the manoeuvre and provide advice on how to improve technique. Common problems and pitfalls include the following.
- Inadequate or incomplete inhalation (to total lung capacity)
- Lack of 'blast effort' during exhalation
- Incomplete emptying of lungs to residual volume (RV) (common in COPD where patients often require longer than the recommended 12 seconds to reach RV)
- An additional breath inwards during the expiratory manoeuvre
- Poor mouthpiece seal (leaks underestimate FEV$_1$ and FVC)
- A slow start to the expiratory manoeuvre (doing so underestimates FEV$_1$)
- Exhaling through the nose
- Coughing
- Poor posture (e.g. leaning excessively forwards or backwards)

## Contraindications to spirometry

Few absolute contraindications to performing spirometry exist. Table 4.4 provides a summary of circumstances where caution is advised.

## Infection control

Precautions are necessary to minimise cross-infection between patients via the spirometer and mouthpiece. Barrier filters and disposable mouthpieces significantly reduce the risks of infection and help protect equipment from exhaled secretions. A new filter should be used for each patient. Manufacturer guidelines should be referred to when cleaning and sterilising equipment.

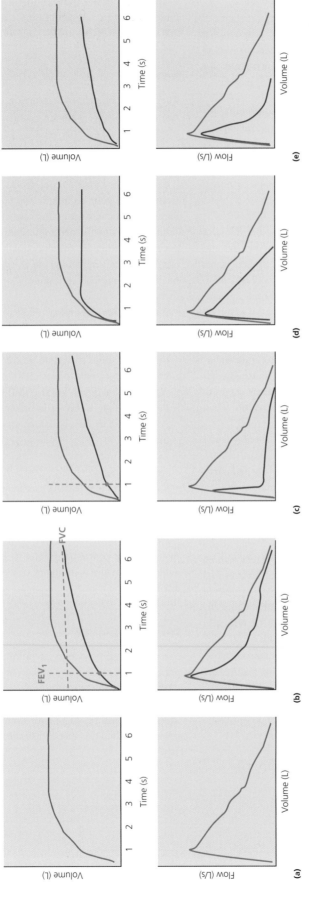

**Figure 4.5** (a) A normal volume/time curve should rise rapidly and smoothly, and in healthy individuals, plateau within 3–4 seconds. A normal flow/volume curve will have a rapid rise to maximal expiratory flow (peak flow) followed by an almost linear uniform decline in flow until all air is exhaled, giving a triangular appearance. (b) Typical volume/time and flow/volume curves in airflow obstruction. Note the reduced forced expiratory volume in 1 second ($FEV_1$) and reduced forced vital capacity (FVC) (indicated in green) in the patient compared to the normal curve. FVC is only recorded for 6 seconds; a longer duration may be required to reach plateau in volume in a patient such as this. A concave dip in the flow/volume curve is evident, which becomes more marked with increasing obstruction. (c) Typical volume/time and flow/volume curves in more severe airflow obstruction. Note that both the $FEV_1$ and FVC are reduced below normal curve (although the former more than the latter). $FEV_1$ (shown in green) is less than in (b). Due to loss of airway elasticity, airways collapse during forced exhalation and a characteristic sudden fall in flow occurs after maximal expiratory flow is reached – a so-called steeple curve. With increasing degrees of airflow obstruction, it takes longer to completely exhale (i.e. reach residual volume) – sometimes up to 15 seconds – and the upward slope (gradient) of the volume/time curve is less and a longer time is taken to reach plateau. (d) Typical volume/time and flow/volume curves with a restrictive ventilatory defect. The shape of the flow/volume curve is normal but a reduction in lung volume is apparent which shifts the FVC point to the left compared with the predicted curve. Note that both the $FEV_1$ and FVC can be proportionally reduced or the $FEV_1$ can be affected to a lesser extent, leading the FEVR to be normal or above normal. (e) Typical volume/time and flow/volume curves with a mixed obstructive and restrictive ventilatory defect. Note that both the $FEV_1$ and FVC are disproportionately reduced.

**Table 4.3** Classification of the severity of airway obstruction according to the National Institute for Health and Care Excellence, American Thoracic Society/European Respiratory Society and Global Initiative for Chronic Obstructive Lung Disease.

| Postbronchodilator FEVR | FEV₁ % predicted | Categorisation of degree of airflow obstruction |
|---|---|---|
| <0.7 | ≥80% | GOLD stage 1 – Mild (providing symptoms are present) |
| <0.7 | 50–79% | GOLD stage 2 – Moderate |
| <0.7 | 30–49% | GOLD stage 3 – Severe |
| <0.7 | <30% | GOLD stage 4 – Very severe |

$FEV_1$, forced expiratory volume in 1 second; FEVR, forced expiratory volume in 1 second ($FEV_1$)/forced vital capacity (FVC) ratio.

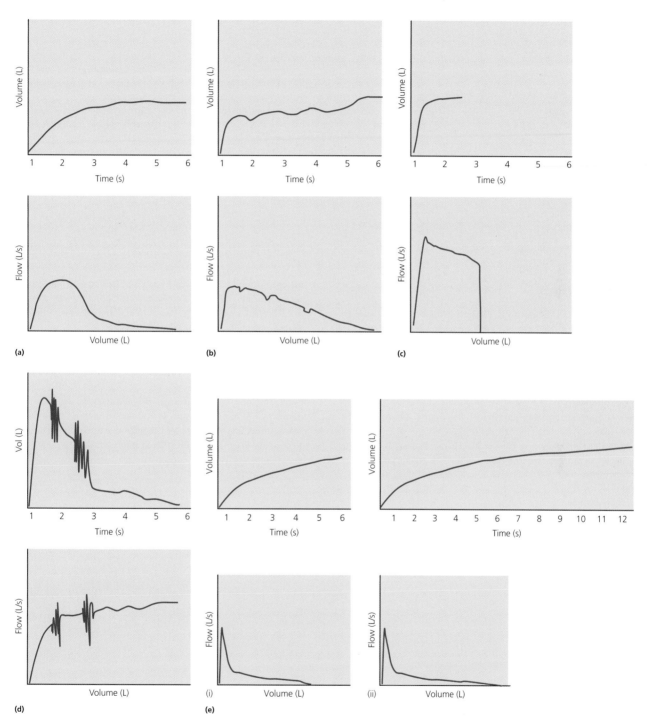

**Figure 4.6** (a) *Problem:* Poor spirometry trace due to a 'slow' start. An adequate duration (6 seconds) is evident and a plateau reached, meaning that VC is probably accurate but $FEV_1$ and peak flow are likely to be underestimated. *Solution:* Repeat the test and encourage a maximal effort at the initial 'blast'. Ensure patient has taken a maximal inspiration prior to the start of the FVC manoeuvre. (b) *Problem:* Poor spirometry trace due to inconsistent/suboptimal effort and a slow start; expiratory flow is interrupted (usually by cough or inhaling then continuing to breathe out). *Solution:* Repeat test and advise the patient to continue to 'breathe out' in one continuous breath. (c) *Problem:* Poor spirometry trace due to an 'early finish'; patient has stopped exhaling after about 2 seconds, before RV is reached: a good effort initially occurs but a plateau is not reached, duration less than 6 seconds and FVC will be underestimated. *Solution:* Advise the patient to 'blow out' until 'lungs are empty'. (d) *Problem:* Cough interrupting expiratory flow. *Solution:* Repeat the test once cough has settled. (e) *Problem:* No plateau. If no plateau is reached in 6 seconds, as in (i) repeat the test and advise patient to continue to 'breathe out' for 12 seconds (or as long as possible). If plateau still not achieved (as in ii), this should be noted when presenting the FVC value. In spirometers that only measure 6 seconds, this can be termed $FEV_6$ (forced expiratory value in 6 seconds).

**Table 4.4** Summary of contraindications and the main reasons to avoid testing.

| Contraindication | Reason to avoid lung function testing* | Recommendation |
|---|---|---|
| Thoracic/abdominal surgery | Rupture site of injury, avoid pain, discomfort | Relative |
| Brain, eye, ear, ENT surgery | Rupture site of injury, avoid pain, discomfort | Relative |
| Pneumothorax | Worsen pneumothorax, avoid discomfort and pain | Relative |
| Myocardial infarction | Induce further infarction leading to cardiac arrest | Absolute/relative |
| Ascending aortic aneurysm | Rupture of aneurysm, catastrophic/fatal event | Absolute/relative |
| Haemoptysis | Pulmonary emboli or myocardial infarction | Relative |
| Pulmonary embolism | Death, hypoxia leading to respiratory failure | Absolute/relative |
| Acute diarrhoea | Discomfort, embarrassment, infection risk | Relative |
| Angina | May lead to cardiac arrest in severe cases, discomfort | Absolute/relative |
| Severe hypertension (systolic >200 mmHg, diastolic >120 mmHg) | Risk of blackout/collapse, rupture of cerebral blood vessels, etc. | Measure blood pressure before tests if suspected |
| Confused/demented patients | Lung function tests are volitional and need patient co-operation | Balance need for test against difficult in obtaining/accuracy of results |
| Patient discomfort | Vomiting, diarrhoea, cold sores, common cold | Wait until main symptoms abate |
| Infection control issue | Contagious infections (norovirus, tuberculosis, influenza) | Wait until main symptoms abate |

* Sometimes the risk may be necessary as a preoperative assessment for life-saving surgery.
Recommendation: absolute, lung function testing should be avoided in most cases; relative, judge each case on its merits.
ENT, ear, nose and throat.
Reproduced with permission from Cooper BG. *Thorax* 2011; **66**: 714–723.

# Further reading

Bolton CE, Ionescu AA, Edwards PH, Faulkner TA, Edwards SM, Shale DJ. Attaining a correct diagnosis of COPD in general practice. *Respiratory Medicine* 2005; **99**: 4939e.

Cooper BG. An update on contraindications for lung function testing. *Thorax* 2011; **66**: 714–723.

Kaminsky DA, Marcy TW, Bachand M, Irvin CG. Knowledge and use of office spirometry for the detection of chronic obstructive pulmonary disease by primary care physicians. *Respiratory Care* 2005; **50**: 1639–1648.

Levy M, Quanjer PH, Booker R, Cooper BG, Holmes S, Small I. Diagnostic spirometry in primary care. Proposed standards for general practice compliant with American Thoracic Society and European Respiratory Society recommendations. *Primary Care Respiratory Journal* 2009; **18**: 130–147.

Miller MR, Hankinson JATS, Brusasco V et al. Standardisation of spirometry. *European Respiratory Journal* 2005; **26**: 319–338.

Quanjer PH, Stanojevic S, Cole TJ et al. ERS Global Lung Function Initiative. Multi-ethnic reference values for spirometry for the 3-95-yr age range: the Global Lung Function 2012 equations. *European Respiratory Journal* 2012; **40**: 1324–1343.

www.ers-education.org/guidelines/global-lung-function-initiative.aspx

Vogelmeier CF, Criner GJ, Martinez FJ et al. Global Strategy for the Diagnosis, Management, and Prevention of Chronic Obstructive Lung Disease 2017 Report. *Eur Respir J* 2017; **49**: 1700214 [https://doi.org/10.1183/13993003.00214-2017].

# CHAPTER 5

# Smoking Cessation

*Sanjay Agrawal[1] and John R. Britton[2]*

[1]Institute of Lung Health, Respiratory Biomedical Research Unit, Glenfield Hospital, Leicester, UK
[2]UK Centre for Tobacco and Alcohol Studies, University of Nottingham, Nottingham, UK *and* City Hospital, Nottingham, UK

---

### OVERVIEW

- Smoking is the biggest avoidable cause of chronic obstructive pulmonary disease (COPD) in developed countries.
- Smoking cessation is the only intervention which has a sustained and significant effect on the natural history of COPD.
- Preventing smoking uptake and promoting smoking cessation are the most effective means of preventing COPD and reducing rates of progression in those with the condition.
- Smoking cessation is the most important treatment for COPD.
- All healthcare workers should encourage individuals to quit smoking at every available opportunity and support those who are willing to try.
- Most smokers want to quit smoking but are addicted to nicotine; several attempts are usually required to successfully quit.
- Smoking cessation is much more likely to be successful if a combination of behavioural support with nicotine replacement therapy, varenicline or bupropion is used.
- Electronic cigarettes may have an important role to play in preventing harm among smokers who feel they are unable or unwilling to quit all nicotine use; they can be useful in helping individuals to quit or reduce the number of cigarettes smoked.
- Electronic cigarettes are likely to be much less harmful than tobacco cigarettes, but long-term safety data are not available.

---

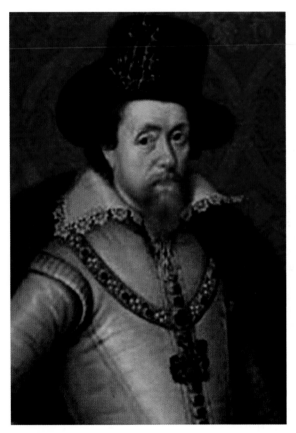

**Figure 5.1** King James I of England.

Smoking was introduced into the United Kingdom in the late 16th century. Shortly afterwards, the son of Mary Queen of Scots, King James I of England, was the first monarch to implement a tax on tobacco use (Figure 5.1). He also published his famous *Counterblaste to tobacco* in 1604 in which he reflected on his dislike of the 'precious stink' and commented that:

> *Smoking is a custom loathsome to the eye, hateful to the nose, harmful to the brain, dangerous to the lungs, and in the black, stinking fume thereof nearest resembling the horrible Stygian smoke of the pit that is bottomless.*

## Who smokes and effects of cigarette smoking

In developed countries, over 80% of individuals with COPD have smoked in the past or are current smokers, while the majority of those with COPD are from less wealthy sections of society. The proportion of the UK adult population who smoke cigarettes has fallen by more than a half in the last 40 years, although this is not the case for those on low incomes (Figures 5.2–5.6). Cigarette smoking varies regionally,

---

Proportion (%) who smoke cigarettes

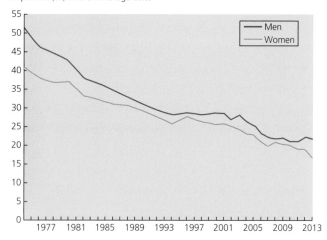

**Figure 5.2** Proportion of population who smoke cigarettes, by sex, Great Britain 1974–2013. Source: Office for National Statistics licensed under Open Government Licence v.3.0. Reproduced with permission.

and is higher among the unemployed, younger individuals, those working in routine and manual occupations and those with lower level educational qualifications, while more males than females smoke. Smokers with COPD often have mental health disorders, including anxiety and depression; the prevalence of smoking in such individuals has remained similar over many decades.

Most smokers with COPD start smoking in adolescence. Children from households in which there are smokers are up to three times more likely to start smoking. Reducing the uptake of smoking in children by limiting their exposure to adults who smoke, and 'denormalising' tobacco use, are therefore likely to lower the number of children who develop COPD as adults.

As well as being the biggest single preventable cause of COPD leading to exacerbations and premature death, smoking (which exposes individuals to the toxic effects of more than 4000 chemicals and carcinogens present in tobacco smoke) also causes or influences the progression of many other diseases and conditions (Table 5.1). Very often, patients with COPD will have more than one smoking-related condition. Helping smokers with COPD to quit smoking

Proportion (%) who smoke cigarettes

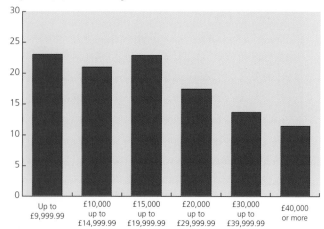

**Figure 5.3** Proportion who smoke cigarettes, by income band, Great Britain, 2013. Source: Office for National Statistics licensed under Open Government Licence v.3.0. Reproduced with permission.

Proportion (%) who smoke cigarettes

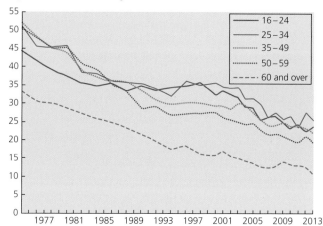

**Figure 5.4** Proportion who smoke cigarettes, by age, Great Britain, 1974–2013. Source: Office for National Statistics licensed under Open Government Licence v.3.0. Reproduced with permission.

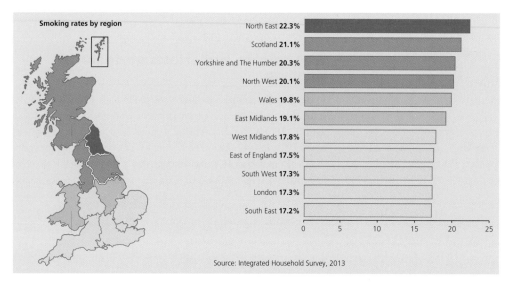

**Figure 5.5** Differences in rates of smoking within Great Britain. Source: Office for National Statistics licensed under Open Government Licence v.3.0. Reproduced with permission.

**Change in cigarette smoking habits over time**
Great Britain 1974–2013

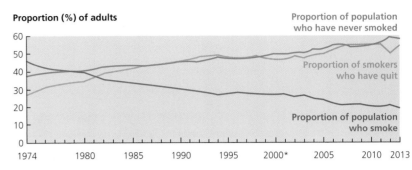

**Figure 5.6** Cigarette smokers as a proportion of the population fell by over 50% between 1974 and 2013. Source: Office for National Statistics licensed under Open Government Licence v.3.0. Reproduced with permission.

Source: Adults Smoking Habits in Great Britain, 2013
*Estimates prior to 2000 are unweighted

**Table 5.1** Cancers, chronic diseases and miscellaneous conditions caused or adversely influenced by cigarette smoking.

| Cancers | Chronic diseases/ conditions | Miscellaneous conditions/associations |
|---|---|---|
| Lung | Ischaemic heart disease | Respiratory tract infections |
| Oropharyngeal | Hypertension | Complications of diabetes |
| Oesophagus | Cerebrovascular disease | Reduced fertility and impotence |
| Bladder | Peripheral vascular disease | Premature ageing |
| Stomach | Age-related macular degeneration | Increased skin wrinkling |
| Pancreatic | Cataracts | Persistent symptoms of asthma |
| Kidney | Chronic obstructive pulmonary disease | Ectopic pregnancy/ miscarriage/stillbirth |
| Cervix | Dementia | Prematurity/low birth weight babies |
| Liver | Osteoporosis | Risks of exposing others to second-hand smoke Increased risk of pneumonia |

therefore offers patients, children, families, healthcare providers and society significant rewards.

## The psychology of addiction

Seventy percent of smokers wish to quit and take an average of 6–7 attempts to successfully do so. Addiction to smoking tobacco is due to nicotine, together with behavioural, environmental and physical cues, for example smoking after meals, outside a bar or restaurant, the physical nature of holding a cigarette and the direct impact on the throat with inhaling.

Nicotine acts on receptors in the brain to release dopamine, which in turn creates a rewarding affect. However, approximately 4–12 hours after smoking a cigarette, regular smokers experience uncomfortable withdrawal symptoms including irritability, anxiety, nervousness and cravings, which in turn perpetuate the desire to use another cigarette in order to relieve symptoms. Although nicotine is the key component in tobacco addiction, it does not cause major health problems in conventional cigarette smokers; rather, it is the tar and other chemicals that accompany nicotine in

tobacco smoke that cause almost all the harm. Individuals with COPD tend to be more addicted to nicotine than other groups of patients and find it harder to quit and relapse more frequently, despite the same desire to stop smoking.

The difficulty in stopping smoking is directly related to the addictive nature of nicotine use rather than apathy. Key criteria for addiction are:
- continual use despite knowledge of harmful consequences
- cravings during abstinence
- failure of attempts to stop
- withdrawal symptoms during abstinence.

## Smoking cessation as a treatment for COPD

Society at large, many individuals with COPD and healthcare workers may consider smoking cessation to be a lifestyle choice rather than a treatment for COPD (in the same way that drugs and pulmonary rehabilitation are treatments for COPD). As with these other treatments, quitting smoking leads to immediate and longer term benefits including less breathlessness, cough, wheeze, improved appetite, fewer exacerbations, fewer admissions to hospitals, necessity for fewer drugs and slower rate of decline in lung function (Figure 5.7). Smoking cessation should be considered a standard part of COPD treatment pathways in primary care, secondary care

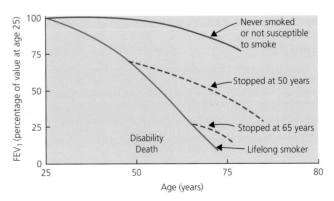

**Figure 5.7** Beneficial effects of smoking cessation occur at any age. FEV$_1$, forced expiratory volume in 1 second. Reproduced from Hogg JC. Pathophysiology of airflow limitation in chronic obstructive pulmonary disease. *Lancet* 2004; **364**: 709–721, with permission from Elsevier.

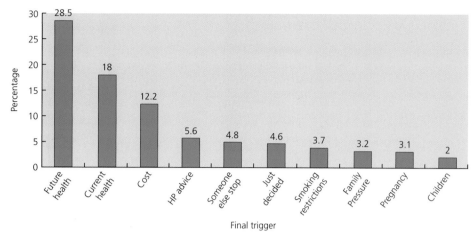

**Figure 5.8** Triggers reported as prompting the most recent quit attempt. HP, health professional. Reproduced with permission from Vangeli E, West R. Sociodemographic differences in triggers to quit smoking: findings from a national survey. *Tobacco Control* 2008; **17**: 410–415.

and social services. All healthcare professionals can play a vital role and can exert a major influence on individuals making a quit attempt (Figure 5.8).

## Helping people to quit smoking

The best way to help individuals with COPD to quit smoking is to refer them to a stop smoking service. Doing so allows trained professionals to explore the most suitable pharmacological adjuncts tailored for the individual and provide behavioural support and follow-up. Stop smoking services are four times more likely to succeed in helping patients quit, versus making a quit attempt on their own.

### Individual training

Those working in healthcare sectors (such as pharmacists, nurses, doctors, therapists and clerical staff) can help patients with COPD to quit smoking. Patients expect to be offered help and support from healthcare staff to help them quit, although many staff members do not have the confidence or knowledge of how to help. The '3 As' offers a simple and practical method to recall how to offer help to smokers (Box 5.1).

---

**Box 5.1 Ensure that the 3 As of smoking cessation are incorporated routinely when exploring and encouraging quit attempts.**

**Ask** – Ask patients if they smoke and record the answer in the notes
**Advise** – That the best way to quit is to use the local smoking cessation service
**Act** – Make a referral to the local smoking cessation service

---

There are many free online resources that can be accessed to train individuals or groups of staff the National Centre for Smoking Cessation and Training (NCSCT). Many patients will not want to stop smoking when asked initially but may accept the offer

on future occasions. Non-judgemental, empathetic, positive motivational techniques are much more effective for those contemplating a quit attempt than 'negative' language (Box 5.2). Provide written information to all those attempting to quit; this can be accessed through the NCSCT.

---

**Box 5.2 Examples of helpful and unhelpful language when encountering individuals who continue to smoke.**

**Examples of helpful/positive language include:**
'It's not easy thinking about stopping'
'It's great that you're thinking about giving up'
'You've stopped before, so I'm sure you can do it again'

**Examples of unhelpful/negative language include:**
'I've told you before that you have to stop smoking and you haven't'
'You've brought this on yourself'
'You should have stopped years ago'
'I can't believe you still haven't stopped'

---

## Healthcare systems

Healthcare staff may work in a variety of settings, e.g. hospitals, general practitioner surgeries, mental health institutions and pharmacies, where there may not be systems in place to support smokers with COPD in quit attempts. The key components to setting up a service in any organisation include:

- having a local 'champion' to lead service development; this can be any healthcare worker and is not dependent on seniority or profession
- implementing a referral pathway to the local stop smoking service or having internal specialist stop smoking advisors
- regularly training staff in the organisation to use the '3 As'
- measuring the number of smokers who are identified and supported to make a quit attempt, to help monitor effectiveness and make changes to the service.

Several national guidelines and quality standards exist to guide indidvuals who want to develop or improve smoking cessation services in their organisation, provided by the National Institute for Health and Care Excellence (NICE), NCSCT and British Thoracic Society.

## Smoking cessation pharmacotherapy
### Nicotine replacement therapy

Nicotine replacement therapy (NRT) is the most commonly used smoking cessation drug therapy and increases the chances of quitting by about 40% (nicotine gum) to 100% (nasal spray). NRT exerts its effects by replacing the supply of nicotine to the individual (thereby reducing craving) without exposure to the toxic components of cigarettes. Many smokers incorrectly believe that nicotine is toxic.

Nicotine replacement therapy is available in many different formulations (Box 5.3). Although some forms of NRT (gum, inhalator delivery, nasal spray or lozenges) deliver nicotine more quickly than others (transdermal patches), all deliver a lower total dose, and deliver it to the brain more slowly than a cigarette. Discuss and offer individuals a choice of different formulations of NRT. Using combination therapy with a transdermal patch to provide continuous background nicotine and a more rapidly acting product (lozenge, gum, inhalator or nasal spray) to use in advance of regular cigarette times and other times of particular craving is helpful. In those with relative contraindications (such as acute cardiovascular disease or pregnancy), it may be prudent to use lower doses of relatively short-acting preparations. Relatively light smokers (<10 cigarettes per day), or those who wait longer than an hour before their first cigarette of the day, may also be better advised to use a short-acting product in advance of their regular cigarettes or at times of craving.

Treatment is generally recommended for 10–12 weeks but smokers may continue to use NRT for longer if they feel they need it. There is no evidence to suggest that gradual withdrawal of NRT is better than abrupt withdrawal, although the former method is usually preferable. NRT products are generally well tolerated and side effects relatively minor. Cautions to NRT use are all relative and should always be overridden if the likely alternative is that the individual will relapse into smoking.

Nicotine replacement therapy may be continued beyond 12 weeks in those smokers who are not able or ready to stop using tobacco altogether as part of a 'cutting down to quit' approach.

## Bupropion

Bupropion has similar efficacy to NRT in improving quit rates (Box 5.4). It is an antidepressant but its effect on smoking cessation is independent of this property, and may be due to effects on noradrenaline and dopamine neurotransmission. Bupropion helps prevent weight gain which often occurs with smoking cessation. The most important adverse effect recognised with bupropion is an association with convulsions; the drug is therefore contraindicated in those with a history of epilepsy and seizures. Bupropion should not generally be prescribed in individuals with other risk factors for seizures and some drugs – such as antidepressants, antimalarials, antipsychotics, quinolones and theophylline – which can lower the seizure threshold.

---

Box 5.3 **Some important prescribing points for NRT.**

- Adverse effects
  - Nausea
  - Headache
  - Unpleasant taste
  - Hiccoughs and indigestion
  - Sore throat
  - Nose bleeds
  - Palpitations
  - Dizziness
  - Insomnia
  - Nasal irritation (spray)
- Cautions and contraindications
  - Hyperthyroidism
  - Diabetes mellitus
  - Renal and hepatic impairment
  - Gastritis and peptic ulcer disease
  - Peripheral vascular disease
  - Skin disorders (patches)
  - Avoid nasal spray when driving or operating machinery (sneezing, watering eyes)
  - Severe cardiovascular disease (arrhythmias, post myocardial infarction)
  - Recent stroke
  - Pregnancy
  - Breastfeeding

---

Box 5.4 **Some important prescribing points for bupropion.**

- Adverse effects
  - Dry mouth
  - Gastrointestinal disturbance
  - Taste disturbance
  - Anxiety
  - Dizziness
  - Depression
  - Headache
  - Reduced concentration and impairment of skilled task performance
  - Insomnia
  - Tremor
  - Fever
  - Itch
  - Rash
  - Sweating
- Cautions and contraindications
  - Pregnancy and breastfeeding
  - Acute alcohol withdrawal
  - Acute benzodiazepine withdrawal
  - Elderly
  - Predisposition to seizures
  - Drugs which lower the seizure threshold
  - History of head trauma
  - Hepatic cirrhosis
  - Bipolar and eating disorder
  - Central nervous system tumours
  - Dose reduction in renal and liver function impairment

Unlike NRT, which is usually started at the same time as quitting smoking, it is recommended that bupropion is commenced in advance of the quit date, by 1 or 2 weeks. Treatment is usually continued for 8 weeks. There is no clear evidence that combining bupropion with NRT confers any further advantage in quit rates; doing so can lead to hypertension and insomnia.

### Varenicline

Varenicline is a partial nicotine agonist, which also blocks nicotine receptors from stimulation by free nicotine. It is an effective smoking cessation treatment which increases the likelihood of quitting by a factor of about 2.3, and is slightly more effective than NRT or bupropion. There is no evidence that combining varenicline with other drug treatments is any more effective than varenicline alone (Box 5.5).

---

Box 5.5 **Some important prescribing points for varenicline.**

- Adverse effects
  - Gastrointestinal disturbance
  - Dry mouth
  - Taste disturbance
  - Headache
  - Drowsiness
  - Dizziness
  - Sleep disturbance and abnormal dreams
- Cautions and contraindications
  - Pregnancy and breastfeeding
  - Predisposition to seizures
  - Cardiovascular disease
  - Suicidal thoughts
  - Depression and psychiatric illness
  - Renal function impairment

---

As for bupropion, start varenicline a week prior to the planned quit day, with increasing doses over the first few days to try and prevent the nausea that some users experience. Depression and suicidal ideation in association with varenicline have been reported, so advise users to stop the drug immediately if they notice any decline in mood.

## Harm reduction

Many individuals with COPD do not wish to consider, or else are not ready or confident enough to try quitting cigarette smoking but would consider reducing their tobacco use. Of those who do reduce their consumption, significant health benefits including reduced breathlessness, cough and exacerbations are likely to occur, while they are also more likely to subsequently quit completely. It is therefore worth encouraging smokers with COPD to consider cutting down if they are initially unwilling to quit. Also encourage such individuals to consider switching, partially or completely, to an alternative source of nicotine. This can include licensed nicotine replacement products or electronic cigarettes (e-cigarettes).

## Electronic cigarettes

Electronic cigarettes were first developed in China around 2003 and became available in the UK and Europe several years later. They are devices that heat a liquid (usually comprising propylene glycol and glycerol) with nicotine (with or without the addition of flavouring) stored in a disposable or refillable cartridge or reservoir. E-cigarettes consist of a battery, atomiser and liquid containing nicotine and generate a smoke-like aerosol (vapour) that the user inhales (or vapes) (Figures 5.9–5.11). Since the vapour typically contains nicotine without most of the toxins associated with conventional cigarettes, many individuals

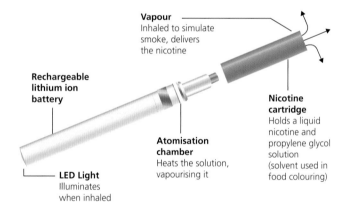

**Vapour**
Inhaled to simulate smoke, delivers the nicotine

**Rechargeable lithium ion battery**

**Nicotine cartridge**
Holds a liquid nicotine and propylene glycol solution (solvent used in food colouring)

**Atomisation chamber**
Heats the solution, vapourising it

**LED Light**
Illuminates when inhaled

**Figure 5.9** Illustration of the typical components of a 'first-generation' e-cigarette.

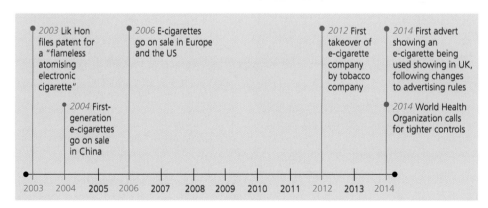

2003 Lik Hon files patent for a "flameless atomising electronic cigarette"

2004 First-generation e-cigarettes go on sale in China

2006 E-cigarettes go on sale in Europe and the US

2012 First takeover of e-cigarette company by tobacco company

2014 First advert showing an e-cigarette being used showing in UK, following changes to advertising rules

2014 World Health Organization calls for tighter controls

2003  2004  2005  2006  2007  2008  2009  2010  2011  2012  2013  2014

**Figure 5.10** Key moments in the growth of the e-cigarette market. Source: Office for National Statistics licensed under Open Government Licence v.3.0. Reproduced with permission.

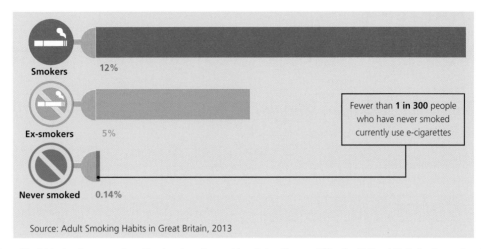

Source: Adult Smoking Habits in Great Britain, 2013

**Figure 5.11** Proportion of individuals who use e-cigarettes, by cigarette smoking status. Source: Office for National Statistics licensed under Open Government Licence v.3.0. Reproduced with permission.

**Table 5.2** Possible advantages and disadvantages of e-cigarettes.

| Advantages | Disadvantages |
| --- | --- |
| Reduces health harms versus use of conventional cigarettes | Long-term health effects unknown |
| Improves smoking quit rates plus reducing number of cigarettes consumed | Confusion among smokers, the general public, media and health professionals about relative risks and benefits |
| Contributes to financial benefits of quitting smoking | Costs (start-up and recurring) |
| Often more acceptable to the general public than other forms of NRT | Could introduce never smokers to nicotine |
| Supports temporary abstinence when tobacco cannot be used to reduce nicotine withdrawal symptoms | May encourage underuse of other forms of NRT or smoking cessation drugs |
| | 'Renormalisation' of smoking |

NRT, nicotine replacement therapy.

use e-cigarettes to provide nicotine replacement as part of a quit attempt or to reduce their tobacco use.

In the UK, the use of e-cigarettes increased 10-fold between 2010 and 2015 with approximately 2.6 million current users. Around 1 in 20 adults in the UK use e-cigarettes, and of these, almost all are either exclusively smokers (60%) or ex-smokers (40%). Their increasing popularity may be partly due to a combination of their chemical, behavioural, ritualistic and sensory similarities to conventional cigarettes; such similarities obviously are not mirrored by other forms of NRT or drugs. E-cigarette use among long-term ex-smokers is considerably lower than among recent ex-smokers and use in never smokers is very low.

Many different models of e-cigarettes exist, which can appear very different to the 'first generation'. They generally deliver different nicotine strengths and flavourings, with users having the ability to choose their preferences in terms of nicotine strength and flavour. There is no evidence that e-cigarette use (or exposure to second-hand vaping) causes major harm in the short term and they are unlikely to be anywhere near as harmful as long-term cigarette use, although long-term safety data are not available. Since e-cigarettes are not 'advised' for never smokers (but only for smokers or former smokers as an alternative to conventional cigarettes or to prevent smoking relapse), any risk should be relative. A Cochrane review of only two studies demonstrated that using an e-cigarette containing nicotine increased the chances of stopping smoking in the long term and that doing so also helped more individuals reduce the amount they smoked by at least half (versus using an e-cigarette without nicotine) (Table 5.2). Electronic cigarettes should therefore be encouraged as a substitute for tobacco cigarettes in smokers who find them more helpful or more acceptable to licensed pharmacotherapies.

## Further reading

McRobbie H, Bullen C, Hartmann-Boyce J, Hajek P. Electronic cigarettes for smoking cessation and reduction. *Cochrane Database of Systematic Reviews* 2014; **12**: CD010216.

www.smokinginengland.info (Smokers toolkit study)

www.ash.org.uk (Action for Smoking on Health (ASH))

www.ncsct.org.uk (National Centre for Smoking Cessation and Training (NCSCT))

www.brit-thoracic.org.uk/document-library/clinical-information/smoking-cessation/bts-recommendations-for-smoking-cessation-services/

www.hqip.org.uk/public/cms/253/625/19/443/COPD%20National%20audit%20-%20organisational%20report%20-%202014.pdf?realName=REYSAO.pdf

www.nice.org.uk/guidance/ph48

www.gov.uk/government/uploads/system/uploads/attachment_data/file/311887/Ecigarettes_report.pdf

www.gov.uk/government/publications/e-cigarettes-an-evidence-update

# CHAPTER 6

# Non-pharmacological Management

*Waleed Salih and Stuart Schembri*

Ninewells Hospital and Medical School, Dundee, UK

---

## OVERVIEW

- The overall aims of chronic obstructive pulmonary disease (COPD) management are multiple and vary according to the individual patient.
- The multidisciplinary team plays an important role in the overall management of patients with COPD.
- Non-pharmacological strategies play a vital role in the management of COPD although they are often given less resource and importance when compared to drugs.
- Complete smoking cessation represents the most important non-pharmacological strategy in symptom reduction and preventing progression.
- Consider pulmonary rehabilitation in all patients; key components are education and graded exercise.
- Pulmonary rehabilitation is associated with improvements in quality of life and exercise capacity, but has no effect on lung function or exacerbation frequency.
- Consider vaccination for influenza and pneumonia in most patients with COPD.
- Arrange professional nutritional advice in underweight and overweight patients.
- Anxiety and depression often co-exist in patients with COPD.

---

Box 6.1 **Some of the main overall treatment aims of COPD.**

- Reduce symptoms.
- Reduce exacerbations.
- Improve lung function.
- Improve exercise tolerance.
- Improve health-related quality of life.
- Provide care tailored to the patient's needs.
- Provide a treatment regime which minimises the risk and frequency of drug-related adverse effects.
- Reduce mortality.
- Prevent or slow down disease progression.

---

## Aims of management

Overall aims in chronic obstructive pulmonary disease (COPD) management are multiple and varied (Box 6.1). Despite significant advancements in pharmacological treatment of COPD, drugs in isolation are unable to facilitate optimal outcomes. While drugs have a significant impact upon important endpoints in clinical trials, they are often prescribed incorrectly and inappropriately, while many patients have suboptimal inhaler technique and poor adherence. Non-pharmacological strategies and multidisciplinary team input, incorporating a broad spectrum of professionals from both primary and secondary care, are therefore increasingly important in overall management and confer benefits complementary to drug use. Many healthcare professionals of varying disciplines can greatly assist patients with the medical, physical, domestic, psychological and social limitations posed by severe breathlessness to function successfully in the community. In some hospitals, dedicated multidisciplinary team meetings take place to address the specific needs of individual patients, most commonly those at the severe end of the disease spectrum (Figure 6.1). When faced with a patient with COPD of any severity, tailor different management strategies to the individual's particular needs (Figure 6.2).

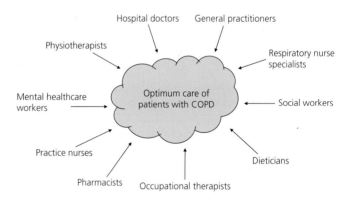

**Figure 6.1** Multidisciplinary team input is required for most patients with COPD.

---

*ABC of COPD*, Third Edition. Edited by Graeme P. Currie.

© 2017 John Wiley & Sons Ltd. Published 2017 by John Wiley & Sons Ltd.

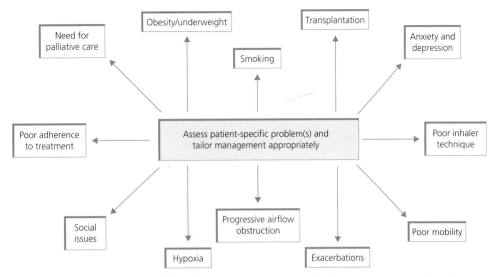

**Figure 6.2** An individualised approach to treatment should be explored when encountering patients with chronic obstructive pulmonary disease of any severity.

## Smoking cessation

Smoking cessation is discussed in detail in Chapter 5. Encouragement to quit underpins the successful management of COPD of all stages. Use every clinical encounter to identify those who continue to smoke cigarettes and offer advice on appropriate quitting methods.

## Pulmonary rehabilitation

Pulmonary rehabilitation is a multidisciplinary intervention aimed at reducing symptoms of COPD and increasing physical activity, thereby improving overall quality of life. The National Institute for Health and Care Excellence (NICE) recommends that it should be offered to symptomatic patients and those who have recently been admitted to hospital with an exacerbation of COPD. The effect of pulmonary rehabilitation declines over time so consider maintenance programmes (when available locally).

### Format

Many healthcare professionals can be involved in the delivery of pulmonary rehabilitation and may include doctors, nurses, respiratory therapists, physiotherapists, occupational therapists, dieticians, nutritionists, psychologists and social workers. There is no standard description of a pulmonary rehabilitation programme but key components usually include graded physical training and education. Pulmonary rehabilitation is helpful in breaking the self-perpetuating vicious circle that patients with COPD frequently encounter (Figure 6.3). Other factors such as immobility, hypoxia, malnutrition, increased oxidative stress and systemic inflammation may all contribute to skeletal muscle atrophy and in turn reduce exercise capacity and heighten fatigue.

Pulmonary rehabilitation is usually delivered to a group of patients, rather than on an individual basis. However, an individualised approach (within the group) is crucial in its success. The duration and intensity of the initial rehabilitation programme required

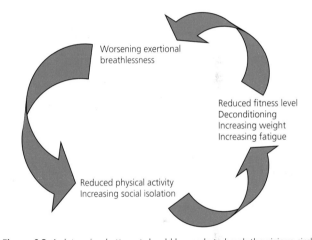

**Figure 6.3** A determined attempt should be made to break the vicious circle of worsening breathlessness, reduced physical activity and deconditioning.

for optimal results are not firmly established, but a minimum length of 6–8 weeks is frequently recommended. Longer programmes may be associated with better outcomes.

### Graded exercise

Comprehensive exercise training, including upper and lower extremity endurance training and strength training, is an essential component of pulmonary rehabilitation. Exercise training is based on general principles of intensity (higher intensity produces greater results), specificity (only those muscles trained show an effect) and reversibility (cessation of regular training results in a decrease in training effect). Strength training is an important component of exercise training and may facilitate additional benefits. Maximising bronchodilation, interval training (i.e. alternating high and low intensities) and oxygen supplementation may facilitate higher intensity exercise training in some patients.

Lower extremity training generally consists of treadmill walking or stationary cycling. Most centres use treadmill walking, given its ease of performance and familiarity to patients. Both high- and low-intensity training programmes have been shown to benefit patients with COPD. Duration, frequency and intensity of training should be tailored to each patient. Individuals should undergo exercise training at as high a level as possible. Patients should undergo at least 20–30 minutes of exercise during each session and perform this at least three times per week, including outwith the rehabilitation sessions. Start the exercise at an intensity level of 60–70% of the patient's predetermined maximum symptom-limited capacity. The duration of exercise should be increased followed by the intensity once preset goals have been met.

Strength training is also an important component of the exercise training programme and may increase muscle strength and mass, increase exercise capacity and improve performance of activities of daily living. Upper extremity training in pulmonary rehabilitation has been shown to increase work capacity of the trained limb and also result in a decrease in oxygen required to perform the same amount of work.

In recent years, other exercise modalities beyond endurance and strength training have been studied. Examples include the following.

### Inspiratory muscle training

As a consequence of COPD, strength and endurance of the diaphragm can be reduced and this contributes to hypercapnia, dyspnoea and reduced walking capacity. Inspiratory muscle training may enhance the dysfunction of the diaphragm and improve some of its consequent burden. The most commonly used inspiratory muscle training method involves 'threshold loading' devices. These generally have a spring-loaded valve requiring the patient to inhale strongly enough to open the valve and to breathe in against an individualised load. In appropriate patients, the addition of inspiratory muscle training to a general exercise training programme can result in improved inspiratory muscle strength and endurance, functional exercise capacity, dyspnoea and quality of life.

### Neuromuscular electrical stimulation

During neuromuscular electrical stimulation (NMES), muscles are stimulated electronically via adhesive electrodes placed on the skin. Most exercise protocols aim for the muscles of the thigh and the calf muscle. The most consistent finding of NMES training in COPD is a 20–30% gain in quadriceps strength.

### Whole-body vibration training

During whole-body vibration training, subjects exercise on a vibrating platform that produces sinusoidal oscillations. Some evidence has demonstrated that whole-body vibration training results in improvements of similar magnitude in terms of exercise capacity, muscle force and quality of life versus conventional strength training.

### Education

Self-management education is an integral component of pulmonary rehabilitation. It promotes self-efficacy and encourages active participation in healthcare. Self-management education has been shown to be highly effective in improving health status and reducing healthcare utilisation. It is usually provided in small group settings and on an individual basis. An initial evaluation helps determine educational needs, which are then reassessed during the course of the programme. Discussions about advance directives are an important part of self-management education, as is counselling about early recognition and treatment of COPD exacerbations. Many other useful techniques can be taught during pulmonary rehabilitation and these may help in reducing symptoms during periods of increased activity or an exacerbation (Table 6.1, Figures 6.4, 6.5).

### Outcomes

Proven and clinically significant benefits of pulmonary rehabilitation include:

- improvements in exercise performance
- better overall health status
- reduction in breathlessness
- reduction in use of healthcare services (decreased hospital admissions)
- reduction in mortality.

There are no data to indicate a reduction in exacerbation frequency or improvement in lung function. However, a Cochrane review demonstrated that pulmonary rehabilitation improved quality of life as measured by both the Chronic Respiratory Questionnaire (CRQ) and St George's Respiratory Questionnaire (SGRQ). Statistically significant improvements in all domains measured by these questionnaires were observed, while improvements larger than the minimal clinically important difference were found in scores for dyspnoea, fatigue, emotional function and mastery in the CRQ and in all domains of the SGRQ. The established benefits of pulmonary rehabilitation are more pronounced in those at the 'highest risk' or, in other words, those who have recently experienced an exacerbation. In a Cochrane review of such patients, significant reductions in hospital admissions and mortality were also noted. Moreover, unlike pharmacological approaches, pulmonary rehabilitation is not associated with adverse effects, although resources, sufficient money, a convenient and accessible location and enthusiastic local lead are all prerequisites.

**Table 6.1** Different techniques which may reduce breathlessness and allow more efficient ventilation.

| Technique | Instruction and effects |
| --- | --- |
| Pursed lip breathing | May reduce respiratory rate and aid recovery during periods of increased activity |
| Relaxed, slower, deeper breathing | May allow more effective ventilation during exertion and avoid rapid shallow breathing |
| Paced breathing | Timing inhalation and exhalation with every other breath may help reduce symptoms during activity |
| Positioning | Passive fixing of the shoulder girdle (for example, elbows resting on a table or ledge) may reduce breathlessness. Patients should also be encouraged to adopt a forward lean sitting position |
| Energy conservation technique | Home adaptations (such as a handrail) or sitting to perform household chores |
| Exhalation on effort | Advise patients to exhale when they perform an activity (such as standing up, lifting the arms) |

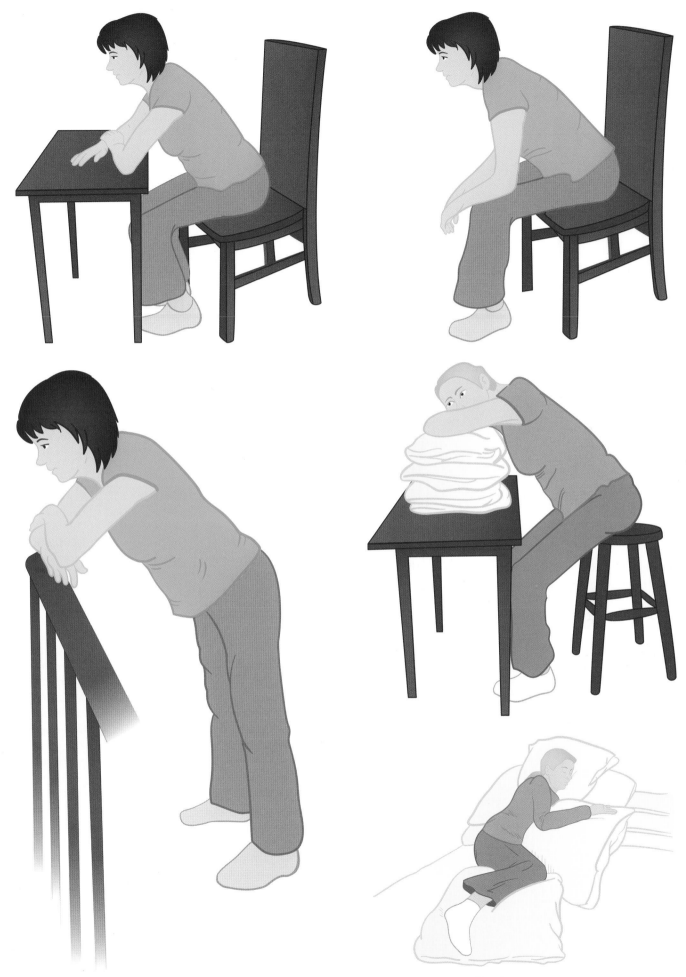

**Figure 6.4** Encourage patients to adopt different positions which use less energy and may help reduce work of breathing.

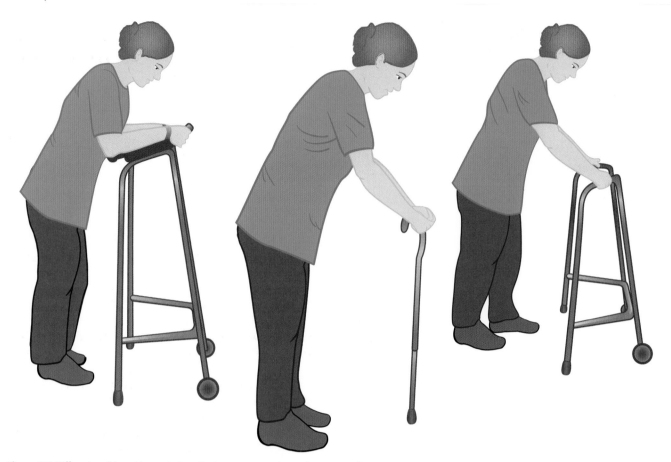

**Figure 6.5** Different walking aids may help patients conserve energy and promote safer movement.

## Nutrition

Many patients with COPD are underweight and malnourished. It is clear that being underweight is a poor prognostic sign in COPD. It is also evident that malnutrition is at least in part associated with the severity of airflow obstruction. The causes of cachexia in patients with COPD are multifactorial and include decreased oral intake (sometimes linked to being too breathless to eat), effects of increased work of breathing due to abnormal respiratory mechanics, and chronic systemic inflammation. Active nutritional supplementation in undernourished patients with COPD can lead to weight gain, improvements in respiratory muscle function and exercise performance. Beneficial effects have been observed when nutritional supplementation is proposed alone or as an adjunct to exercise training.

Patients with COPD may have difficulty following advice that simply consists of being told to 'eat more'. Education regarding the calorific value of different food types, with emphasis on the need to increase quantities of fat in the diet, can be helpful. Simple suggestions include using full-fat milk rather than skimmed or semi-skimmed, adding powdered milk to liquid milk to increase calorific content without increasing volume and having 'cream' soups rather than broths. A Cochrane review demonstrated that supplementation promotes significant weight gain among malnourished patients with COPD; this was associated with significant improvements in respiratory muscle strength and quality of life.

At the opposite end of the spectrum, some individuals with COPD may be overweight.

## Immunisation

### Influenza vaccination

Influenza is a global threat. Rates of serious illness due to influenza viruses are highest among the elderly and those with chronic conditions. Complications of influenza infection include viral pneumonia, secondary bacterial pneumonia and other secondary bacterial infections such as bronchitis, sinusitis and otitis media (Figure 6.6). Healthy individuals usually recover within 1 week but influenza infection in patients with underlying medical conditions such as COPD is associated with higher risks and may lead to hospital admission and death. Although the evidence is inconclusive, influenza vaccine may reduce hospital admissions and mortality from COPD.

Current guidelines recommend that all patients with COPD receive influenza vaccination annually. Quadrivalent vaccines offering protection against two strains of influenza, A and B, are available annually based on the predicted circulating strain that year. The only absolute contraindication to influenza vaccination is severe allergy (anaphylaxis) to eggs. Newer influenza vaccines that do not use embryonated eggs are currently in development. Other recent developments in this area include high-dose vaccine specifically at people 65 years of age and older although this is not currently available in the UK.

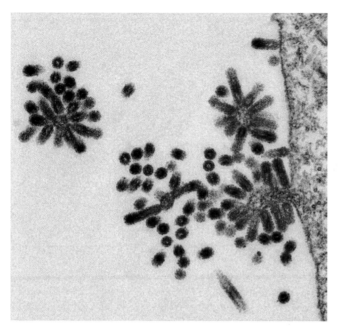

**Figure 6.6** Electron micrograph showing influenza viruses (*red*) budding from a host cell. Reproduced with permission from sciencephoto.com.

Few randomized studies have looked at the effect of influenza vaccination specifically in COPD. A Cochrane review in 2006, updated in 2010, suggested that influenza vaccination reduced COPD exacerbations and this is supported by many observational studies, including some that have also shown a mortality benefit.

## Pneumococcal vaccination

The pneumococcal polysaccharide vaccine (PPV) has been found to be effective in the prevention of pneumococcal pneumonia and bacteraemia in previously healthy young individuals, and also in certain groups of patients at high risk of developing pneumococcal infection. The vaccine contains capsular polysaccharide antigens from the 23 most dominant serotypes among clinical isolates of *S. pneumoniae*, accounting for approximately 80–90% of overall invasive infections in the adult population. These antigens induce type-specific antibodies (by a T-cell-independent mechanism) that enhance opsonisation, phagocytosis and killing of pneumococci by phagocytic cells.

Pneumococcal polysaccharide vaccine is recommended for patients with COPD 65 years and older. This vaccine has been shown to reduce the incidence of community-acquired pneumonia in COPD patients younger than age 65 with forced expiratory volume in 1 second <40% predicted. Revaccination (5–10 years after prime dose) should be considered in those persons who received PPV-23 before 65 years of age. It must not be forgotten, however, that PPV-23 provides incomplete protection, it does not elicit long-lasting immunity and no anamnestic effect occurs at revaccination.

Newer conjugate vaccines protecting against different *S. pneumoniae* subtypes are available but their recommended use in the UK is currently limited to a paediatric population.

In conclusion, influenza and pneumococcal infection are major causes of morbidity and mortality in those with COPD. Influenza vaccination clearly reduces acute exacerbations of COPD

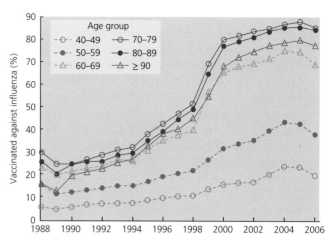

**Figure 6.7** Trends in vaccination rates against influenza in patients aged >40years with chronic obstructive pulmonary disease. Figure reproduced with permission from Schembri S, Morant S, Winter JH, MacDonald TM. Influenza but not pneumococcal vaccination protects against all-cause mortality in patients with COPD. *Thorax* 2009; **64**: 567–572. Reproduced with permission of BMJ Publishing Group Ltd.

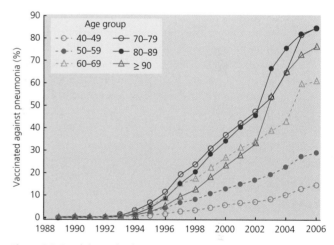

**Figure 6.8** Trends in vaccination rates against pneumonia in patients aged >40years with chronic obstructive pulmonary disease. Figure reproduced with permission from Schembri S, Morant S, Winter JH, MacDonald TM. Influenza but not pneumococcal vaccination protects against all-cause mortality in patients with COPD. *Thorax* 2009; **64**: 567–572. Reproduced with permission of BMJ Publishing Group Ltd.

(Figures 6.7, 6.8). In addition, it may reduce hospitalizations and mortality, although data are inconclusive. Pneumococcal vaccination reduces invasive pneumococcal disease, but there are few data demonstrating concrete clinically significant health benefits in patients with COPD. Vaccination with both influenza and pneumococcal vaccine may produce an additive protective effect. There are major efforts under way to develop more effective pneumococcal vaccines.

## Anxiety and depression

Anxiety and depression often co-exist in patients with COPD and are underrecognised and undertreated. Moreover, concomitant depression may be associated with poorer quality of life, reduced survival, persistent smoking, higher hospital admission rates and more symptoms. The presence of anxiety or depression in patients with COPD has also been directly associated with the severity of airflow obstruction. All this suggests that interventions that reduce anxiety and depression should be considered where necessary. These conditions are likely to be multifactorial in origin, with social isolation, persistent symptoms and inability to easily participate in activities of daily living all playing a role.

Clinical features suggestive of an anxiety or depressive disorder should be positively sought in all patients with COPD; one simple way of assessing this is by the Hospital Anxiety and Depression Scale (Box 6.2). Tiredness, low energy, weight loss and poor sleep are fairly non-specific and often occur in both COPD and depression. If anxiety or depression is likely to be present, consider drug treatments, although robust evidence suggesting a major beneficial effect is lacking. In depression, tricyclic antidepressants or selective serotonin reuptake inhibitors should be considered, whereas in anxiety, selective serotonin reuptake inhibitors and benzodiazepines are options. If benzodiazepines are prescribed, clinicians should be vigilant for respiratory depression and oversedation. An aggressive attempt to optimise lung function and treat significant hypoxaemia should also be undertaken in these patients. Psychotherapy, including cognitive behavioural therapy, has been applied in patients in an attempt to minimise the undesirable cognitive processes associated with breathlessness. Such therapy aims to reduce anxiety by stopping the dyspnoea–anxiety–dyspnoea cycle. Pulmonary rehabilitation may help reduce anxiety in COPD patients.

---

Box 6.2 **Hospital Anxiety and Depression Scale.**

**Anxiety**
- I feel tense or wound up
  *Most of the time – 3, a lot of the time – 2, from time to time – 1, not at all – 0*
- I get a sort of frightened feeling as if something awful is going to happen
  *Definitely and badly – 3, yes, but not too badly – 2, a little – 1, not at all – 0*
- Worrying thoughts go through my mind
  *Very definitely – 3, yes, but not too badly – 2, a little – 1, not at all – 0*
- I can sit at ease and feel relaxed
  *Definitely – 0, usually – 1, not often – 2, not at all – 3*
- I get a sort of frightened feeling like butterflies in the stomach
  *Not at all – 0, occasionally – 1, quite often – 2, very often – 3*
- I feel restless as if I have to be on the move
  *Very much indeed – 3, quite a lot – 2, not very much – 1, not at all – 0*
- I get sudden feelings of panic
  *Very often indeed – 3, quite often – 2, not very often – 1, not at all – 0*

**Depression**
- I look forward with enjoyment to things
  *As much as I ever did – 0, rather less than I used to – 1, definitely less than I used to – 2, hardly at all – 3*
- I have lost interest in my appearance
  *Definitely – 3, I take not so much care as I should – 2, I may not take quite as much care – 1, I take as much care as ever – 0*
- I still enjoy the things I used to enjoy
  *Definitely as much – 0, not quite so much – 1, only a little – 2, hardly at all – 3*
- I can laugh and see the funny side of things
  *As much as I always could – 0, not quite so much – 1, definitely not so much – 2, not at all – 3*
- I feel cheerful
  *Not at all – 3, not often – 2, sometimes – 1, most of the time – 0*
- I feel as if I am slowed down
  *Nearly all the time – 3, very often – 2, sometimes – 1, not at all – 0*
- I can enjoy a good book, the radio or a TV programme
  *Often – 0, sometimes – 1, not often – 2, seldom – 3*

Scoring is based on a 4-point scale (0–3). A score of 0–7 is normal, 8–10 borderline and 11–21 suggests moderate-to-severe anxiety or depression.

---

## Acknowledgment

The authors would like to thank Charlie Dear, Department of Medical Illustration, Aberdeen Royal Infirmary for artwork.

## Further reading

Ferreira IM, Brooks D, White J, Goldstein R. Nutritional supplementation for stable chronic obstructive pulmonary disease. *Cochrane Database of Systematic Reviews* 2012; **12**: CD000998.

McCarthy B, Casey D, Devane D, Murphy K, Murphy E, Lacasse Y. Pulmonary rehabilitation for chronic obstructive pulmonary disease. *Cochrane Database of Systematic Reviews* 2015; **2**: CD003793.

Mikkelsen RL, Middelboe T, Pisinger C, Stage KB. Anxiety and depression in patients with chronic obstructive pulmonary disease (COPD). *A review*. *Nordic Journal of Psychiatry* 2004; **58**: 65–70.

Puhan MA, Gimeno-Santos E, Scharplatz M, Troosters T, Walters EH, Steurer J. Pulmonary rehabilitation following exacerbations of chronic obstructive pulmonary disease. *Cochrane Database of Systematic Reviews* 2011; **10**: CD005305.

Wongsurakiat P, Maranetra KN, Wasi C, Kositanont U, Dejsomritrutai W, Charoenratanakul S. Acute respiratory illness in patients with COPD and the effectiveness of influenza vaccination: a randomized controlled study. *Chest* 2004; **125**: 2011–2020.

# CHAPTER 7

# Pharmacological Management I – Inhaled Treatment

*Graeme P. Currie*[1] *and Brian J. Lipworth*[2]

[1] Aberdeen Royal Infirmary, Aberdeen, UK
[2] Scottish Centre for Respiratory Research, Ninewells Hospital and Medical School, Dundee, UK

## OVERVIEW

- Prescribe a short-acting bronchodilator (short-acting $\beta_2$-agonist (SABA) or short-acting muscarinic antagonist (SAMA)) for as-required relief of symptoms in all patients with chronic obstructive pulmonary disease (COPD).

- For patients in (Global Initiative for Chronic Obstructive Lung Disease (GOLD) group A) (few symptoms and infrequent exacerbations) use a SABA or SAMA alone.

- For patients in GOLD group B (persistent symptoms and infrequent exacerbations) use monotherapy with either a long-acting muscarinic antagonist (LAMA) or long-acting $\beta_2$-agonist (LABA). Prescribe a LAMA/LABA combination inhaler if symptoms persist despite LAMA or LABA as monotherapy.

- For patients in GOLD group C (with few symptoms and frequent exacerbations) despite monotherapy, use a combination inhaler containing either LAMA/LABA or inhaled corticosteroid (ICS)/LABA (if $FEV_1 < 50\%$ predicted).

- For patients in GOLD group D with persistent symptoms and frequent exacerbations despite LAMA/LABA use triple therapy with an ICS/LABA combination plus LAMA (if $FEV_1 < 50\%$ predicted).

- Inhaled corticosteroids play no role as monotherapy in COPD; only prescribe them in a single inhaler device also containing a LABA.

- Reduction in exacerbations with ICS given as dual or triple therapy is greater in patients with blood eosinophils >2%.

- Guidelines emphasise the importance of de-escalating treatment (eg from ICS/LAMA/LABA to LAMA/LABA), if therapeutic trials have been unsuccessful.

Chronic obstructive pulmonary disease (COPD) is a heterogeneous condition and all patients should be regarded as individuals. This is apparent not only in terms of presentation, natural history, symptoms, disability and frequency of exacerbations but also in response to treatment. Guidelines indicate that the stepwise titration of pharmacological therapy in COPD should usually be based around (NICE 2010; Vogelmeier et al. 2017):

- extent of airflow obstruction based on postbronchodilator forced expiratory volume in 1 second ($FEV_1$) % predicted
- severity of symptoms (usually breathlessness)
- frequency of annual exacerbations (including hospital admissions)
- the composite Global Initiative for Chronic Obstructive Lung Disease (GOLD) classification of disease severity based around lung function (stages 1–4) plus symptoms and exacerbations (A–D) (Box 7.1).

---

Box 7.1 **Characterisation of patients according to the Global Initiative for Chronic Obstructive Lung Disease (Vogelmeier et al. 2017). Patients should be classified as belonging to groups A, B, C or D depending on exacerbation frequency and symptoms (based on the modified Medical Research Council dyspnoea scale (mMRC) and COPD assessment test (CAT); see Chapter 3). Patients can be characterised further depending on lung function (GOLD stages 1, 2, 3, and 4 denotes $FEV_1$% predicted ≥80%, 50–79%, 30–49% and 30% respectively).**

- GOLD A: few symptoms (mMRC <2, CAT <10) and <2 exacerbations annually
- GOLD B: persistent symptoms (mMRC ≥2, CAT ≥10) and <2 exacerbations annually
- GOLD C: few symptoms and ≥2 exacerbations annually
- GOLD D: persistent symptoms and ≥2 exacerbations annually

---

## Physiological effects of inhaled bronchodilators

Air trapping, which manifests clinically as hyperinflation, is frequently found in patients with advanced COPD; this places the respiratory muscles at a mechanical disadvantage. During exercise, air trapping increases even further, which in turn perpetuates the mechanical disadvantage experienced at rest (Figure 7.1).

Inhaled bronchodilators reduce measures of air trapping at rest and on exercise (static and dynamic hyperinflation), which may

---

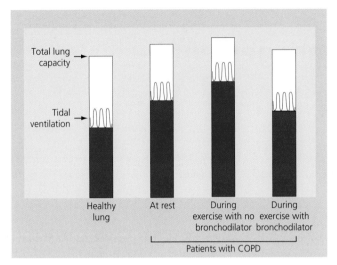

**Figure 7.1** Patients with COPD often have pulmonary hyperinflation with an increased functional residual capacity (*purple*) and decreased inspiratory capacity (*white*). This increases the volume at which tidal breathing (*oscillating line*) occurs and places the muscles of respiration at mechanical disadvantage. Hyperinflation worsens with exercise and therefore reduces exercise tolerance (dynamic hyperinflation). Inhaled bronchodilators reduce dynamic hyperinflation, in addition to hyperinflation at rest, thereby reducing the work of breathing and increasing exercise tolerance.

occur without significant changes in $FEV_1$ but result in improvements in forced vital capacity. As COPD is largely an irreversible condition, relying solely on outcome measures such as lung function may result in potentially important beneficial effects being missed upon parameters such as lung volumes, quality of life and exacerbation frequency.

## Short-acting bronchodilators

Short-acting $\beta_2$-agonists (SABAs), such as salbutamol and terbutaline, act directly upon bronchial smooth muscle to dilate the airways (Table 7.1). Drugs within this class reduce breathlessness and improve lung function (Sestini et al. 2002).

Ipratropium is the main short-acting muscarinic antagonist (SAMA) and offsets high-resting bronchomotor vagally induced tone to dilate the airways. It has been shown in some studies to reduce breathlessness and improve lung function and quality of life (Appleton et al. 2006).

Prescribe a short-acting inhaled bronchodilator (SABA or SAMA) for as-required relief of symptoms in all patients with COPD. There are no major differences in responses to either class and no great benefit from combining both classes or from using

**Table 7.1** Properties of short acting $\beta_2$-agonists.

| Bronchodilator class | Drug | Onset of action | Peak effect | Duration |
|---|---|---|---|---|
| Short-acting $\beta_2$-agonist | Salbutamol/ terbutaline | 5 minutes | 60–90 minutes | 4–6 hours |
| Short-acting anticholinergic | Ipratropium | 15 minutes | 30–60 minutes | 3–5 hours |

them on a regular daily basis (NICE 2010; Vogelmeier et al. 2017). Patients using a long-acting muscarinic antagonist (LAMA) should *not* be prescribed ipratropium, but instead use a SABA for acute symptom relief.

In patients with minimal symptoms, preserved lung function ($FEV_1 > 80\%$ predicted) and few (if any) exacerbations, prescribe a SAMA or SABA as monotherapy (without the need for any other inhaled treatment) for as-required use (GOLD A) (NICE 2010; Vogelmeier et al. 2017).

## Long-acting bronchodilators

In COPD, the two classes of inhaled long-acting bronchodilators available are LAMAs and long-acting $\beta_2$-agonists (LABAs) (Table 7.2). As well as being available for use as the individual drug, some long-acting bronchodilators have been formulated to deliver both classes of drug (LAMA and LABA) in a single combination inhaler device. Both LAMAs and LABAs generally improve lung function, reduce exacerbations and improve quality of life.

Guidelines indicate that long-acting bronchodilators should be given initially as monotherapy in symptomatic patients in GOLD group B. If symptoms persist thereafter, both classes of long-acting bronchodilator may be used in either two separate devices or more conveniently in a combined LAMA/LABA inhaler device. LAMAs and LABAs are usually well tolerated, although adverse effects do occur in some patients (Box 7.2).

---

**Box 7.2 Adverse effects of long-acting bronchodilators.**

- Long-acting $\beta_2$-agonists
  - Tachycardia
  - Palpitation
  - Myocardial ischaemia
  - Peripheral vasodilation
  - Fine tremor
  - Headache
  - Muscle cramps
  - Prolongation of the QT interval
  - Hypokalaemia
  - Feeling of nervousness
  - Paradoxical bronchospasm
  - Sleep disturbance
- Long-acting anticholinergics
  - Dry mouth
  - Nausea
  - Constipation
  - Diarrhoea
  - Cough
  - Headache
  - Tachycardia
  - Acute angle glaucoma
  - Bladder outflow obstruction
  - Paradoxical bronchospasm
  - Blurred vision

**Table 7.2** Characteristics of long-acting bronchodilator monotherapy inhalers.

| Class | Drug | Brand name | Delivery device type | Delivery device name | Dose | Frequency |
|---|---|---|---|---|---|---|
| LAMA | Tiotropium | Spiriva | DPI | Handihaler | 18 µg | Once daily |
| LAMA | Tiotropium | Spiriva | FMI | Respimat | 5 µg | Once daily |
| LAMA | Aclidinium | Eklira | DPI | Genuair | 375 µg | Twice daily |
| LAMA | Glycopyrronium | Seebri | DPI | Breezhaler | 50 µg | Once daily |
| LAMA | Umeclidinium | Incruse | DPI | Ellipta | 55 µg | Once daily |
| LABA | Formoterol | Altimos | pMDI | pMDI | 12 µg | Twice daily |
| LABA | Formoterol | Oxis/Foradil | DPI | Turbohaler/Easyhaler | 12 µg | Twice daily |
| LABA | Salmeterol | Serevent | DPI | Accuhaler | 50 µg | Twice daily |
| LABA | Salmeterol | Serevent | pMDI | pMDI | 50 µg | Twice daily |
| LABA | Indacaterol | Onbrez | DPI | Breezhaler | 150/300 µg | Once daily |
| LABA | Olodaterol | Striverdi | FMI | Respimat | 5 µg | Once daily |

DPI, dry powder inhaler; FMI, fine mist inhaler; LABA, long-acting $\beta_2$-agonist; LAMA, long-acting muscarinic antagonist; pMDI, pressurised metered dose inhaler. Reproduced with permission from Currie GP, Lipworth B. Inhaled treatment for chronic obstructive pulmonary disease: what's new and how does it fit? *Quarterly Journal of Medicine* 2016; **109**: 505–512. Note that Tiotropium DPI is also available as Braltus 10 µg once daily.

## Long-acting muscarinic antagonists

Airflow obstruction in COPD is multifactorial in origin and is in part due to potentially reversible high cholinergic tone. Mechanisms mediated by the vagus nerve are implicated in enhanced submucosal gland secretion in patients with COPD. This knowledge has led to the development of LAMAs such as the once-daily drugs tiotropium, umeclidinium and glycopyrronium, and twice-daily aclidinium.

Three main subtypes ($M_1$, $M_2$ and $M_3$) of muscarinic receptor exist. The activation of both $M_1$ and $M_3$ receptors results in bronchoconstriction whereas the $M_2$ receptor is protective against such an effect and attenuates acetycholine release. All LAMAs are relatively selective for $M_3$ receptors while ipratropium (a SAMA) is non-selective. Blocking $M_2$ receptors with ipratropium may remove the brake from prejunctional acetylcholine release and overcome postjunctional $M_3$ blockade by concurrent use of a LAMA.

Long-acting muscarinic antagonists cause a reduction in resting bronchomotor tone, smooth muscle relaxation and prolonged bronchodilation. They are administered via breath-actuated dry powder inhalers (DPI), while tiotropium is also available as a solution-based multidose Respimat fine mist solution inhaler (FMI).

In a Cochrane review of 22 studies (Karner et al. 2014), tiotropium was associated with a significant improvement in quality of life and reduction in exacerbations compared to placebo. In a further Cochrane review of seven studies (Chong et al. 2012), tiotropium was similar to LABAs in improving quality of life and lung function, although the former was more effective than LABAs in preventing exacerbations and hospital admissions. The mechanism by which tiotropium reduces exacerbations is probably blockage of the proinflammatory effects of acetylcholine rather than classic effects of smooth muscle relaxation. Despite safety concerns with different tiotropium delivery devices, in a randomised controlled trial comparing tiotropium given via DPI and FMI to 17 135 patients with COPD over approximately 2 years, no differences were observed in risk of death, major adverse cardiovascular events or exacerbations (Wise et al. 2013).

In a further study (Tashkin et al. 2008), the effects of add-on tiotropium to all other medication were evaluated over a 4-year period in nearly 6000 patients with $FEV_1 < 70\%$ predicted. Compared to placebo, tiotropium was associated with improvements in lung function, quality of life, mortality and exacerbations, although it failed to reduce the overall rate of decline in $FEV_1$; a subgroup analysis indicated that in patients with less advanced disease (mean $FEV_1$ 59% predicted), tiotropium did slow the rate of lung function decline (Decramer et al. 2009) (Figure 7.2).

## Long-acting $\beta_2$-agonists

Long-acting $\beta_2$-agonists act directly upon $\beta_2$-adrenoceptors, causing smooth muscle to relax and airways to dilate. The two most widely used drugs, formoterol and salmeterol, are given on a twice-daily basis. In contrast to SABAs, both salmeterol and formoterol are relatively lipophilic (fat soluble) and have prolonged receptor occupancy. Factors such as these, as well as exoreceptor binding with salmeterol, may in part explain their prolonged duration of action. Formoterol is a more potent agonist than salmeterol in terms of smooth muscle relaxation, and has a more rapid onset of action. A Cochrane systematic review of 26 trials evaluated effects of LABAs in patients with COPD after treatment of at least 3 months (Kew et al. 2013). It demonstrated that they were associated with improved quality of life and fewer exacerbations compared to placebo, but failed to reduce mortality.

New ultra-LABAs have been developed to be given on a once-daily basis as monotherapy; examples include indacaterol and olodaterol. Another once-daily LABA, vilanterol, is currently only available in combination with the LAMA umeclidinium or with the ICS fluticasone furoate. In the largest meta-analysis of once-daily LABAs across 13 studies (Geake et al. 2015), indacaterol resulted in statistically significant and clinically meaningful improvements in lung function and quality of life compared to placebo. In the same study, lung function improvement was comparable to that of well-established twice-daily LABAs. In a further multicentre study (Decramer et al. 2013), 3444 patients with severe COPD were randomised to receive indacaterol or tiotropium for 1 year. Both

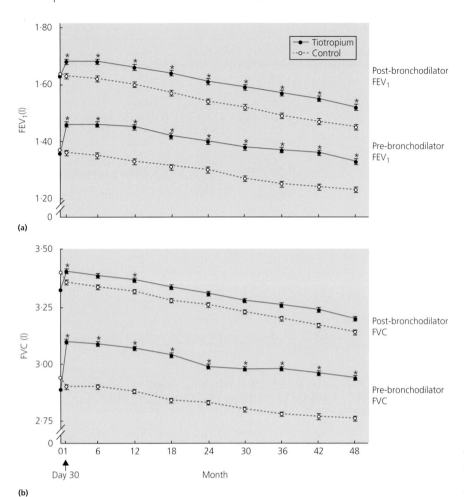

(a)

(b)

**Figure 7.2** Effects of add-on tiotropium on mean pre- and postbronchodilator forced expiratory volume in 1 second ($FEV_1$) (a) and forced vital capacity (FVC) (b) in patients with less advanced COPD. Reproduced from Decramer et al. (2009), with permission of Elsevier.

treatments conferred clinically relevant improvements in lung function at 12 weeks, with indacaterol being non-inferior to tiotropium, while patients receiving tiotropium experienced fewer exacerbations. Bateman et al. combined outcomes of two studies involving more than 3000 patients receiving aclidinium plus formoterol versus the individual constituents and placebo (Bateman et al. 2015). Over 24 weeks, improvements ($p < 0.05$) in symptoms with the combination inhaler versus the LABA and LAMA alone and placebo occurred, with moderate or severe exacerbations significantly reduced with the LAMA/LABA versus placebo (but not monotherapies).

## Long-acting bronchodilator combination inhalers

Several studies have evaluated the effects of different inhalers containing both classes of long-acting bronchodilators (Table 7.3); these have shown superiority compared to each respective monocomponent in terms of $FEV_1$ and symptoms, and in some cases exacerbations and quality of life (Buhl et al. 2015; Moitra et al. 2015; Rodrigo and Neffen 2015; Rodrigo and Plaza 2014). There are no data consistently demonstrating greater all-round superiority of the different combined LAMA/LABA formulations.

**Table 7.3** Characteristics of long-acting bronchodilator combination inhalers.

| Class | Drug | Brand name | Delivery device type | Delivery device name | Dose | Frequency |
|---|---|---|---|---|---|---|
| LAMA/LABA | Aclidinium/Formoterol | Duaklir | DPI | Genuair | 340/12 µg | Twice daily |
| LAMA/LABA | Umeclidinium/Vilanterol | Anoro | DPI | Ellipta | 55/22 µg | Once daily |
| LAMA/LABA | Glycopyrronium/Indacaterol | Ultibro | DPI | Breezhaler | 43/85 µg | Once daily |
| LAMA/LABA | Tiotropium/Olodaterol | Spiolto | FMI | Respimat | 5/5 µg | Once daily |

DPI, dry powder inhaler; FMI, fine mist inhaler; LABA, long-acting $\beta_2$-agonist; LAMA, long-acting muscarinic antagonist; pMDI, pressurised metered dose inhaler. Reproduced with permission from Currie GP, Lipworth B. Inhaled treatment for chronic obstructive pulmonary disease: what's new and how does it fit? *Quarterly Journal of Medicine* 2016; **109**: 505–512. Note that Glycopyrrolate /Formoterol pMDI is also available as Bevespi Aerosphere 18µg/9.6µg twice daily.

The choice of which combination inhaler is prescribed should usually be determined by cost, ease of dosing regimen and patient preference in terms of inhaler device. It is also intuitive that if a patient requires switching from LAMA alone to LAMA/LABA combination, the same device should be used. Using a single dual-component LAMA/LABA inhaler is preferable and usually more cost-effective than using two separate inhalers, while adherence is likely to be better with a single combination inhaler.

## Inhaled corticosteroids

Considerable debate has taken place over the years as to the exact clinical effects of ICS in COPD, whether they should be prescribed, and if so, who should receive them, at what dose, whether they are associated with an increased risk of pneumonia and other serious adverse effects, and if any overall benefits outweigh drawbacks associated with long-term use. Given these contentions, multiple large multicentre studies and meta-analyses have attempted to address the unanswered questions surrounding their use.

Examples of ICS include twice-daily beclomethasone dipropionate, budesonide and fluticasone propionate, although these drugs are only licensed for use when combined with a LABA in a single inhaler device. It is important to note that many patients with COPD – even those with minimal symptoms and mild airflow obstruction – have been (and are currently) treated with ICS as monotherapy. This is despite the relative insensitivity of corticosteroids upon neutrophilic inflammation found in most patients with COPD and paucity of evidence showing significant short- or long-term benefits as monotherapy. Historically, this may be due to clinicians incorrectly extrapolating the beneficial role of anti-inflammatory treatment in asthma to that of COPD, uncertainty as to whether the patient had COPD or asthma plus lack of alternative pharmacological strategies previously available. However, with the introduction and increasingly widespread use of different types of long-acting bronchodilators, it is possible that the prescription of ICS in the future will be directed to individuals most likely to experience benefit.

It is fairly well established that ICS as monotherapy do not have any appreciable impact upon reducing the rate of decline in $FEV_1$ (Figure 7.3) or mortality. In one large study (Burge et al. 2000), add-on 1000 µg/day of fluticasone conferred a 25% reduction in exacerbations, with most benefit observed in patients with mean $FEV_1 < 50\%$ predicted. In other studies, there have been inconsistent effects upon secondary endpoints, with either no or only small improvements in symptoms and quality of life. In a Cochrane meta-analysis evaluating >16 000 individuals (Yang et al. 2012), long-term ICS failed to reduce the decline in $FEV_1$ and no mortality benefit was observed. Treatment was, however, associated with reductions in the mean rate of exacerbations and rate of decline in quality of life; beneficial responses were unable to be predicted by oral steroid response, bronchodilator reversibility or bronchial hyperresponsiveness. In a further study, ICS withdrawal was associated with a 43 mL decline in $FEV_1$ after a year but no impact on exacerbations (see Figure 7.3) (Magnussen et al. 2014). Recent data have suggested that there may be a small subgroup of patients, with so-called asthma COPD overlap syndrome, who may respond better to ICS in

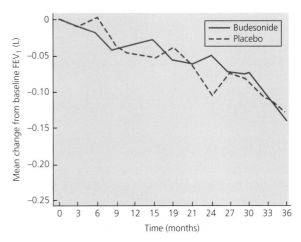

**Figure 7.3** Inhaled corticosteroids have not been shown to influence the rate of decline in lung function in COPD. In this study of patients with mild COPD, no difference in mean change in baseline forced expiratory volume in 1 second ($FEV_1$) between placebo and budesonide was observed over 36 months. Reproduced from Vestbo et al. (1999), with permission of Elsevier.

terms of exacerbation reduction, and can be identified by a raised peripheral blood eosinophil count (Pascoe et al. 2015).

The dose of ICS required to achieve maximal beneficial effect with minimal adverse effect (optimum therapeutic ratio) is uncertain. As a result, combined ICS/LABA inhaler devices all contain ICS of different potency and dose. Current guidelines suggest that ICS should generally be prescribed in patients with $FEV_1 < 50\%$ predicted (in a combination inhaler with a LABA) who experience frequent ($\geq 2$ per year) exacerbations (GOLD C and D).

## Adverse effects of inhaled corticosteroids

Inhaled corticosteroids cause both local and systemic adverse effects. Common local adverse sequelae include oropharyngeal candidiasis and dysphonia. Previous studies have shown that skin bruising occurs more commonly in patients using ICS (Figure 7.4), while variable dose-related effects have been observed in terms of reduction of bone mineral density (osteoporosis) and cortisol (adrenal insufficiency) (Yang et al. 2012).

In the TORCH study with fluticasone propionate (Calverley et al. 2007) and in another study (Dransfield et al. 2013) evaluating fluticasone furoate, an increased risk of pneumonia was found in patients receiving ICS alone and when used in conjunction with a LABA. Other post hoc analysis data have shown the propensity for pneumonia to be greater with fluticasone propionate compared to budesonide (Halpin et al. 2011; Janson et al. 2013; Suissa et al. 2013). In a further study, it was suggested that the association with pneumonia and inhaled corticosteroids may not be a class effect, as across seven trials (including 3801 patients), no increased incidence of pneumonia was observed with budesonide (Sin et al. 2009). Explanations for the possible link between fluticasone and pneumonia have been postulated such as its higher lipophilicity resulting in more prolonged local immune suppression in the lung, altering the lung microbiome in patients with COPD who have impaired mucociliary clearance (Sze et al. 2012). However, in a Cochrane review across 43 studies (Kew and Seniukovich 2014), it

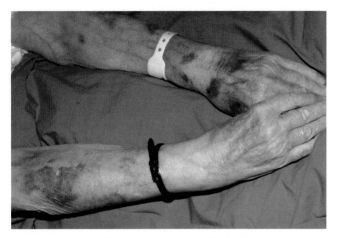

**Figure 7.4** Extensive skin bruising in a patient with COPD using long-term high-dose inhaled corticosteroids.

**Table 7.4** Characteristics of inhaled corticosteroid and long-acting $\beta_2$-agonist combination inhalers.

| Class | Drug | Brand name | Delivery device type | Dose | Frequency |
|---|---|---|---|---|---|
| ICS/LABA | Fluticasone propionate/Salmeterol | Seretide | DPI | 500/50 µg | Twice daily |
| ICS/LABA | Budesonide/Formoterol | Symbicort | DPI | 400/12 µg | Twice daily |
| ICS/LABA | Budesonide/Formoterol | DuoResp Spiromax | DPI | 400/12 µg | Twice daily |
| ICS/LABA | Fluticasone furoate/Vilanterol | Relvar | DPI | 92/22 µg | Once daily |
| ICS/LABA | Beclomethasone/Formoterol | Fostair | pMDI or DPI | 200/12 µg | Twice daily |

DPI, dry powder inhaler; ICS, inhaled corticosteroid; LABA, long-acting $\beta_2$-agonist; pMDI, pressurised metered dose inhaler.
Reproduced with permission from Currie GP, Lipworth B. Inhaled treatment for chronic obstructive pulmonary disease: what's new and how does it fit? *Quarterly Journal of Medicine* 2016; **109**: 505–512. Note that budesonide/formoterol as Symbicort pMDI suspension is also available 400/12 µg twice daily; fluticasone/salmeterol as AirFluSal Forspiro DPI 500/50 µg twice daily; AirDuo RespiClick DPI 232/14 µg twice daily; Aerivio Spiromax DPI 500/50 µg twice daily.

was concluded that budesonide and fluticasone (delivered alone or in combination with a LABA) were associated with increased risk of pneumonia, but neither significantly affected mortality versus controls. In some of the studies highlighted above, 'pneumonia' did not have to be confirmed radiologically, and it is pertinent to emphasise that increased pneumonia events have not been directly linked to an increase in mortality (Marzoratti et al. 2013).

## Combined inhaled corticosteroid plus long-acting $\beta_2$-agonist inhalers

Most studies evaluating LABAs and ICS have shown superiority with the combination product over the single agent alone. For example, in the largest study evaluating this combination of drugs (TORCH) (Calverley et al. 2007), fluticasone propionate plus salmeterol in combination was better than either drug as monotherapy in terms of survival, $FEV_1$, exacerbation frequency and quality of life over a 3-year period. In the same study, the primary endpoint of all-cause mortality with the combination product was not achieved. In studies evaluating the combination of budesonide with formoterol, the proportion of reductions in exacerbations (25%) was similar to the TORCH study with the combination product versus placebo. In most studies evaluating LABAs and ICS in combination in general, the mean $FEV_1$ was <50% predicted. In the study by Wedzicha et al. (2008), the combination of fluticasone plus salmeterol was compared to tiotropium; exacerbation rates were similar in both groups, although pneumonia was more common but mortality lower with the combination treatment. In >3000 patients with COPD (Dransfield et al. 2013), it was demonstrated that the addition of fluticasone furoate to vilanterol resulted in a reduction in moderate and severe exacerbations compared to the vilanterol-only group, but also an increased risk of pneumonia. More recently the FLAME study showed that treatment with LABA/LAMA (Indacaterol/glycopyrronium) was superior to ICS/LABA (fluticasone-salmeterol) on the primary outcome of exacerbations (11% lower), irrespective of blood eosinophil count. Moreover, LABA/LAMA was also superior on trough lung function ($FEV_1$) and quality of life (Wedzicha et al. 2016).

Several different types of combined ICS/LABAs inhalers are available (Table 7.4). Combined ICS/LABA devices are generally indicated when individuals have an $FEV_1 < 50\%$ predicted and ≥2 exacerbations annually. For ICS/LABA combination inhalers, there is currently only one licensed pressurised metered inhaler (pMDI) containing beclomethasone/formoterol. Most patients will require the use of an approved spacer device such as an Aerochamber to obviate co-ordination problems using a pMDI alone and reduce the likelihood of ICS-related local adverse effects. In COPD, budesonide/formoterol and beclomethasone/formoterol are only licensed for fixed dose maintenance therapy (unlike in asthma where these combinations of drugs can be used for relief of symptoms).

## Triple therapy

In advanced symptomatic COPD, many patients are prescribed triple therapy with a combination of a LAMA, LABA and ICS. Currently, no inhaled device contains all three drug classes, and patients need to use a monocomponent LAMA inhaler plus combined ICS/LABA device.

In studies by Tashkin et al. (2008) and Welte et al. (2009), add-on tiotropium to fluticasone plus salmeterol resulted in a reduction in exacerbations in one study but not the other. The GLISTEN study demonstrated significant improvements in $FEV_1$ and quality of life plus reduction in rescue medication use when either tiotropium or glycopyrronium was added to fluticasone plus salmeterol over 3 months (Figure 7.5) (Frith et al. 2015). In a retrospective cohort study (Short et al. 2012), 2853 patients with moderate-to-severe COPD were followed up for 4–5 years, of whom 996 were receiving ICS/LABA and 1857 ICS/LABA/LAMA. Comparing outcomes using triple versus dual therapy, there was a 15% reduction for

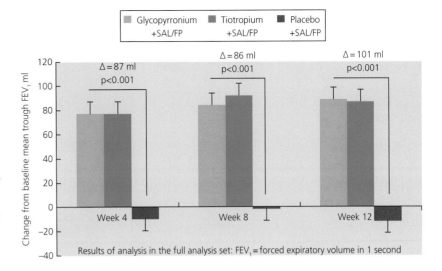

**Figure 7.5** Trough forced expiratory volume in 1 second (FEV$_1$) at weeks 4, 8 and 12 (full analysis set). Comparable outcomes for glycopyrronium versus tiotropium (i.e. non-inferiority) were also demonstrated for all other outcome measures (health status, rescue medication use, nocturnal symptoms and activity performance). FP, fluticasone propionate; SAL, salmeterol. Reproduced with permission from Frith et al. (2015).

hospital admissions, 29% reduction for oral corticosteroid bursts and 26% reduction for all-cause mortality. A further study (analysing overall outcomes of two separate studies across a total of >1000 patients) involving the combination of umeclidinium plus fluticasone furoate/vilanterol (Siler et al. 2015) also supports the use of triple therapy in improving lung function with some improvement in symptom reduction.

More recently, the FULFIL trial over 6 months showed that using a single triple inhaler comprising fluticasone furoate/vilanterol/umecilidinium once daily was superior to a single dual inhaler comprising budesonide/formoterol twice daily on both lung function and exacerbations but not on quality of life (Lipson et al. 2017). In the Trilogy trial comparing a single triple twice daily inhaler comprising beclometasone/formoterol/glycopyrronium verses a single dual twice daily inhaler comprising beclometasone/formoterol, there were also superior improvements in lung function and exacerbations over 12 months (Singh et al. 2016).

It remains to be seen if for patients in GOLD D who fail to respond to LAMA/LAMA single inhaler and who have blood eosinophilia, the use a single triple inhaler will confer benefit.

## Practical considerations

Stripped back to the simplest of forms, inhaled treatment in the management of patients with COPD has four basic pharmacological steps based around a variety of parameters influencing disease severity (Figure 7.6). While this appears at first glance to represent an easy, practical and pragmatic guide by which to escalate treatment, in 'real life' this is unfortunately not always the case. Difficulties arise because of problems such as:

- monocomponent corticosteroids inhalers are not licensed for use in COPD
- no single inhaler device can deliver all the different classes of drug to facilitate both prevention and relief of acute symptoms
- escalating treatment, to include a different class of drug, may involve patients switching inhaler device
- patients will invariably need to correctly recall how (and when) to use different inhaler devices

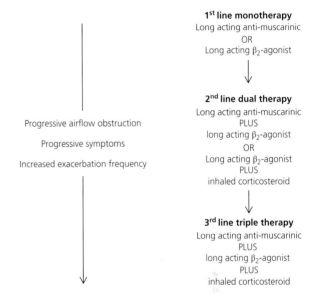

**Figure 7.6** The main pharmacological prescribing steps for inhaled treatment in patients with chronic obstructive pulmonary disease. Reproduced with permission from Currie GP, Lipworth B. Inhaled treatment for chronic obstructive pulmonary disease: what's new and how does it fit? *Quarterly Journal of Medicine* 2016; **109**: 505–512. Note that treatment should be discontinued if a therapeutic trial has been unsuccessful.

- many primary and secondary care prescribing clinicians and nurses are unlikely to have in-depth knowledge of the array of new inhaled drugs and devices currently available.

## Summary of inhaled treatment

The relative effects of the different classes of inhaled drugs used for COPD are shown in Table 7.5. Since airflow obstruction is the universal feature of clinically significant COPD, bronchodilators play an integral role in all stages of disease, while ICS should be reserved for patients with more advanced airflow obstruction and who experience frequent exacerbations (GOLD C and D), especially in those with blood eosinophils >2%. Many new drugs and inhaler devices have been recently introduced to be used as both

**Table 7.5** Relative effects of the main classes of inhaled drugs on important endpoints, both individually and combined, when used in chronic obstructive pulmonary disease.

| Parameter | Monotherapy LAMA | Monotherapy LABA | Monotherapy ICS | LAMA/LABA combination | ICS/LABA combination | ICS/LABA plus LAMA |
|---|---|---|---|---|---|---|
| Symptoms/quality of life | + | + | 0 | ++ | + | ++/+++ |
| Exacerbations | + | + | 0 | ++ | +/++ | ++/+++ |
| Lung function | + | + | 0 | ++/+++ | + | ++/+++ |
| Effect on mortality | 0 | 0 | 0 | 0 | 0 | +/− |
| Rate of lung function decline | 0 | 0 | 0 | 0 | 0 | 0 |

ICS, inhaled corticosteroid; LABA, long-acting $\beta_2$-agonist; LAMA, long-acting muscarinic antagonist.

+, +/− and 0 denote relative magnitude of beneficial effect, equivocal effect or little or no effect respectively.

The efficacy of ICS as ICS/LABA or ICS/LABA/LAMA is relatively greater in patients with "eosinophilic" COPD for reducing exacerbations.

monotherapy and combined with different classes. In addition to tiotropium, new LAMAs include umcledinium, aclidinium and glycopyrronium. As well as being formulated individually, all of these LAMAs have been formulated to be delivered in a single combination inhaler also containing a LABA. In addition to the well-established LABA/ICS inhalers containing formoterol/budesonide and salmeterol/fluticasone, newer combination inhalers containing fluticasone furoate/vilanterol and beclomethasone/formoterol have been introduced.

Guidelines suggest that regular inhaled drugs (alone or in combination) should be given depending on a composite risk assessment based on airflow obstruction ($FEV_1$ % predicted), exacerbation frequency and symptoms (see Box 7.1). If $FEV_1$ is ≥50% predicted, options include a LAMA or LABA alone, or a combination LAMA/LABA single inhaler if symptoms and exacerbations persist. If $FEV_1$ is <50% predicted and symptoms and exacerbations persist, options include dual therapy with a LAMA/LABA combination inhaler, ICS/LABA combination inhaler or triple therapy with ICS/LABA combination plus LAMA (as two separate inhalers), particularly with ICS being used when blood eosinophils exceed >2%. In such circumstances, patients should be made aware of the potential risk of developing side effects including pneumonia and osteoporosis with high ICS doses. For GOLD D patients who are likely to benefit from an ICS moiety, a single triple inhaler comprising either once daily fluticasone furoate/vilanterol/umeclidinium or twice daily becleometasone/formoterol/glycopyrrounium my be better than ICS/LABA. In such patients it remains unclear where a triple inhaler would be superior to LAMA/LABA.

## References

Appleton S, Jones T, Poole P et al. Ipratropium bromide versus short acting beta-2 agonists for stable chronic obstructive pulmonary disease. *Cochrane Database of Systematic Reviews* 2006; **2**: CD001387.

Bateman ED, Chapman KR, Singh D et al. Aclidinium bromide and formoterol fumarate as a fixed-dose combination in COPD: pooled analysis of symptoms and exacerbations from two six-month, multicentre, randomised studies (ACLIFORM and AUGMENT). *Respiratory Research* 2015; **16**: 92.

Buhl R, Gessner C, Schuermann W et al. Efficacy and safety of once-daily QVA149 compared with the free combination of once-daily tiotropium plus twice-daily formoterol in patients with moderate-to-severe COPD (QUANTIFY): a randomised, non-inferiority study. *Thorax* 2015; **70**: 311–319.

Burge PS, Calverley PM, Jones PW, Spencer S, Anderson JA, Maslen TK. Randomised, double blind, placebo controlled study of fluticasone propionate in patients with moderate to severe chronic obstructive pulmonary disease: the ISOLDE trial. *BMJ* 2000; **320**: 1297–1303.

Calverley PM, Anderson JA, Celli B et al. Salmeterol and fluticasone propionate and survival in chronic obstructive pulmonary disease. *New England Journal of Medicine* 2007; **356**: 775–789.

Chong J, Karner C, Poole P. Tiotropium versus long-acting beta-agonists for stable chronic obstructive pulmonary disease. *Cochrane Database of Systematic Reviews* 2012; **9**: CD009157.

Decramer M, Celli B, Kesten S, Lystig T, Mehra S, Tashkin DP. Effect of tiotropium on outcomes in patients with moderate chronic obstructive pulmonary disease (UPLIFT): a prespecified subgroup analysis of a randomised controlled trial. *Lancet* 2009; **374**: 1171–1178.

Decramer ML, Chapman KR, Dahl R et al. Once-daily indacaterol versus tiotropium for patients with severe chronic obstructive pulmonary disease (INVIGORATE): a randomised, blinded, parallel-group study. *Lancet Respiratory Medicine* 2013; **1**: 524–533.

Dransfield MT, Bourbeau J, Jones PW et al. Once-daily inhaled fluticasone furoate and vilanterol versus vilanterol only for prevention of exacerbations of COPD: two replicate double-blind, parallel-group, randomised controlled trials. *Lancet Respiratory Medicine* 2013; **1**: 210–223.

Frith PA, Thompson PJ, Ratnavadivel R et al. Glycopyrronium once-daily significantly improves lung function and health status when combined with salmeterol/fluticasone in patients with COPD: the GLISTEN study, a randomised controlled trial. *Thorax* 2015; **70**: 519–527.

Geake JB, Dabscheck EJ, Wood-Baker R, Cates CJ. Indacaterol, a once-daily beta2-agonist, versus twice-daily beta(2)-agonists or placebo for chronic obstructive pulmonary disease. *Cochrane Database of Systematic Reviews* 2015; **1**: CD010139.

Halpin DM, Gray J, Edwards SJ, Morais J, Singh D. Budesonide/formoterol vs. salmeterol/fluticasone in COPD: a systematic review and adjusted indirect comparison of pneumonia in randomised controlled trials. *International Journal of Clinical Practice* 2011; **65**: 764–774.

Janson C, Larsson K, Lisspers KH et al. Pneumonia and pneumonia related mortality in patients with COPD treated with fixed combinations of inhaled corticosteroid and long acting beta2 agonist: observational matched cohort study (PATHOS). *BMJ* 2013; **346**: f3306.

Karner C, Chong J, Poole P. Tiotropium versus placebo for chronic obstructive pulmonary disease. *Cochrane Database of Systematic Reviews* 2014; **7**: CD009285.

Kew KM, Seniukovich A. Inhaled steroids and risk of pneumonia for chronic obstructive pulmonary disease. *Cochrane Database of Systematic Reviews* 2014; **3**: CD010115.

Kew KM, Mavergames C, Walters JA. Long-acting beta2-agonists for chronic obstructive pulmonary disease. *Cochrane Database of Systematic Reviews* 2013; **10**: CD010177.

Lipson DA, Barnacle H, Birk R, Brealey N, Locantore N, Lomas DA, Ludwig-Sengpiel A, Mohindra R, Tabberer M, Zhu C, Pascoe SJ. FULFIL Trial: Once-Daily Triple Therapy in Patients with Chronic Obstructive Pulmonary Disease. AJRCCM Articles in Press. Published on 04-April-2017 as 10.1164/rccm.201703-0449OC).

Magnussen H, Disse B, Rodriguez-Roisin R et al. Withdrawal of inhaled glucocorticoids and exacerbations of COPD. *New England Journal of Medicine* 2014; **371**: 1285–1294.

Marzoratti L, Iannella HA, Waterer GW. Inhaled corticosteroids and the increased risk of pneumonia. *Therapeutic Advances in Respiratory Disease* 2013; **7**: 225–234.

Moitra S, Bhome AB, Brashier BB. Aclidinium bromide/formoterol fixed-dose combination therapy for COPD: the evidence to date. *Drug Design Development and Therapy* 2015; **9**: 1989–1999.

National Institute for Health and Care Excellence. CG101: Chronic Obstructive Pulmonary Disease. National Clinical Guideline on Management of Chronic Obstructive Pulmonary Disease in Adults in Primary and Secondary Care. 2010. Available at: www.nice.org.uk/guidance/cg101 (accessed 21 February 2017).

Pascoe S, Locantore N, Dransfield MT, Barnes NC, Pavord ID. Blood eosinophil counts, exacerbations, and response to the addition of inhaled fluticasone furoate to vilanterol in patients with chronic obstructive pulmonary disease: a secondary analysis of data from two parallel randomised controlled trials. *Lancet Respiratory Medicine* 2015; **3**: 435–442.

Rodrigo GJ, Neffen H. A systematic review of the efficacy and safety of a fixed-dose combination of umeclidinium and vilanterol for the treatment of COPD. *Chest* 2015; **148**: 397–407.

Rodrigo GJ, Plaza V. Efficacy and safety of a fixed-dose combination of indacaterol and glycopyrronium for the treatment of COPD: a systematic review. *Chest* 2014; **146**: 309–317.

Sestini P, Renzoni E, Robinson S, Poole P, Ram FS. Short-acting beta 2 agonists for stable chronic obstructive pulmonary disease. *Cochrane Database of Systematic Reviews* 2002; **4**: CD001495.

Short PM, Williamson PA, Elder DH, Lipworth SI, Schembri S, Lipworth BJ. The impact of tiotropium on mortality and exacerbations when added to inhaled corticosteroids and long-acting beta-agonist therapy in COPD. *Chest* 2012; **141**: 81–86.

Siler TM, Kerwin E, Sousa AR, Donald A, Ali R, Church A. Efficacy and safety of umeclidinium added to fluticasone furoate/vilanterol in chronic obstructive pulmonary disease: results of two randomized studies. *Respiratory Medicine* 2015; **109**: 1155–1163.

Sin DD, Tashkin D, Zhang X et al. Budesonide and the risk of pneumonia: a meta-analysis of individual patient data. *Lancet* 2009; **374**: 712–719.

Singh D, Papi A, Corradi M, Pavlišov I, Montagna I, Francisco C, Cohuet G, Vezzoli S, Scuri M, Vestbo J. Single inhaler triple therapy versus inhaled corticosteroid plus long-acting β2-agonist therapy for chronic obstructive pulmonary disease (TRILOGY): a double-blind, parallel group, randomised controlled trial. Lancet 2016;388:963-973.

Suissa S, Patenaude V, Lapi F, Ernst P. Inhaled corticosteroids in COPD and the risk of serious pneumonia. *Thorax* 2013; **68**: 1029–1036.

Sze MA, Dimitriu PA, Hayashi S et al. The lung tissue microbiome in chronic obstructive pulmonary disease. *American Journal of Respiratory and Critical Care Medicine* 2012; **185**: 1073–1080.

Tashkin DP, Celli B, Senn S et al. A 4-year trial of tiotropium in chronic obstructive pulmonary disease. *New England Journal of Medicine* 2008; **359**: 1543–1554.

Vestbo J, Sorensen T, Lange P, Brix A, Torre P, Viskum K. Long-term effect of inhaled budesonide in mild and moderate chronic obstructive pulmonary disease: a randomised controlled trial. *Lancet* 1999; **353**: 1819–1823.

Vogelmeier CF, Criner GJ, Martinez FJ et al. Global Strategy for the Diagnosis, Management, and Prevention of Chronic Obstructive Lung Disease 2017 Report. *Eur Respir J* 2017; **49**: 1700214 [https://doi.org/10.1183/13993003.00214-2017].

Wedzicha JA, Banerji D, Chapman KR et al. Indacaterol–Glycopyrronium versus Salmeterol–Fluticasone for COPD. *N Engl J Med* 2016; **374**: 2222–2234.

Wedzicha JA, Calverley PM, Seemungal TA, Hagan G, Ansari Z, Stockley RA. The prevention of chronic obstructive pulmonary disease exacerbations by salmeterol/fluticasone propionate or tiotropium bromide. *American Journal of Respiratory and Critical Care Medicine* 2008; **177**: 19–26.

Welte T, Miravitlles M, Hernandez P et al. Efficacy and tolerability of budesonide/formoterol added to tiotropium in patients with chronic obstructive pulmonary disease. *American Journal of Respiratory and Critical Care Medicine* 2009; **180**: 741–750.

Wise RA, Anzueto A, Cotton D et al. Tiotropium Respimat inhaler and the risk of death in COPD. *New England Journal of Medicine* 2013; **369**: 1491–1501.

Yang IA, Clarke MS, Sim EH, Fong KM. Inhaled corticosteroids for stable chronic obstructive pulmonary disease. *Cochrane Database of Systematic Reviews* 2012; **7**: CD002991.

# CHAPTER 8

# Pharmacological Management II – Oral Treatment

*Graeme P. Currie[1] and Brian J. Lipworth[2]*

[1] Aberdeen Royal Infirmary, Aberdeen, UK
[2] Scottish Centre for Respiratory Research, Ninewells Hospital and Medical School, Dundee, UK

---

## OVERVIEW

- No reliably useful or effective oral bronchodilator without significant adverse effects exists for patients with chronic obstructive pulmonary disease (COPD).

- Theophylline is a non-selective phosphodiesterase inhibitor with weak bronchodilator and anti-inflammatory effects. It has a limited role in the management of stable COPD; low doses may confer benefit by activation of histone deacetylase and may potentiate anti-inflammatory activity of inhaled corticosteroids.

- Selective phosphodiesterase-4 inhibitors have been shown to reduce exacerbations of COPD (especially in those with chronic bronchitis) and produce small improvements in lung function additive to long-acting inhaled bronchodilators; their use is limited by adverse effects such as gastrointestinal upset, headache and weight loss. They can be considered in patients with advanced airflow obstruction, especially those with chronic bronchitis using maximal inhaled therapy.

- No evidence exists indicating that long-term oral corticosteroids are of benefit in COPD; avoid them if possible due to adverse effects.

- The role of mucolytics is not clear, although they may reduce exacerbations in selected patients.

- No evidence exists demonstrating benefit with regular use of mucolytics in patients with COPD using maximal inhaled therapy.

- Long-term macrolide antibiotics may have a role in a minority of patients with advanced COPD who experience frequent infective exacerbations, especially if they have concomitant bronchiectesis; the risk of adverse effects and bacterial resistance requires careful consideration prior to adopting this approach.

- When used for cardiovascular disease, $\beta_1$-selective β-blockers are associated with a reduction in mortality and exacerbations of COPD, probably due to cardioprotective effects. They are not contraindicated in COPD of any severity.

Inhaled treatment forms the cornerstone of pharmacological management in chronic obstructive pulmonary disease (COPD). However, many individuals – especially the elderly, those with cognitive impairment, upper limb musculoskeletal problems such as rheumatoid arthritis and very low inspiratory flow rates – often experience technical difficulties with, and are unable to consistently and successfully use, inhaler devices.

Unfortunately, there are significant unmet needs in terms of effective oral drugs free from troublesome adverse effects available to treat patients on a long-term basis. Although few major advances have been made in this respect over the past few decades, a number of oral drugs can be considered in different circumstances in a selected number of patients.

## Theophylline

Theophylline (Figures 8.1, 8.2) is one of the oldest oral therapeutic agents available for the treatment of COPD (Barnes 2003). It has a chemical structure similar to caffeine, which is also a bronchodilator in large amounts. Theophylline is a non-selective phosphodiesterase (PDE) inhibitor which results in an increase in levels of intracellular cyclic adenosine monophosphate (cAMP) in a variety of cell types and organs (including the lungs).

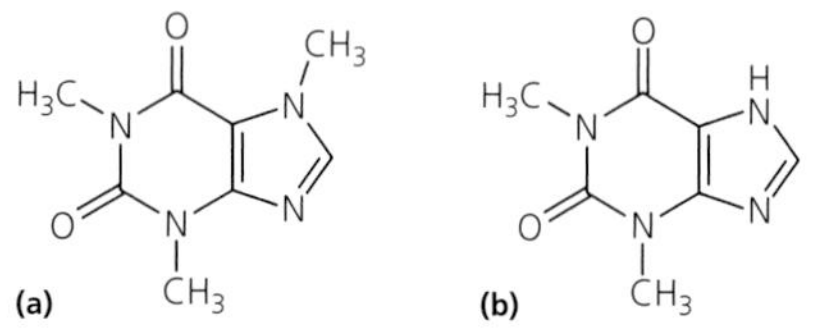

**Figure 8.1** Chemical structures of (a) caffeine and (b) theophylline are similar.

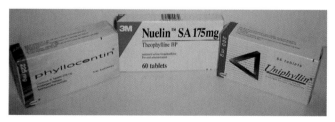

**Figure 8.2** A variety of long-acting theophylline preparations are available and are usually given to patients in modified-release preparations.

---

Increases in cAMP levels are implicated in inhibitory effects upon inflammatory and immunomodulatory cells. One of the end results is that PDE inhibition causes relaxation of smooth muscle and subsequent bronchodilation. However, a number of other potentially beneficial mechanisms of action of theophylline in COPD have been suggested. These include:

- reduction of diaphragmatic muscle fatigue
- increased mucociliary clearance
- respiratory centre stimulation
- inhibition of neutrophilic inflammation
- suppression of inflammatory genes by activation of histone deacetylases
- inhibition of cytokines and other inflammatory cell mediators
- potentiation of anti-inflammatory effects of inhaled corticosteroids at low doses (via increased histone deacetylase activity)
- potentiation of bronchodilator effects of $\beta_2$-agonists.

## Clinical use of theophylline

In recent years, theophylline has been used less extensively because of limited efficacy, narrow therapeutic index, commonly encountered adverse effects, increased use of more effective inhaled bronchodilators and interactions with many other drugs. However, a therapeutic trial of a long-acting theophylline should still be considered in patients with more advanced COPD, especially when symptoms persist despite the use of maximal inhaled treatments or when patients are unable to use inhaler devices.

Various studies have demonstrated that theophylline can result in small benefits in lung function (as reflected by the forced expiratory volume in 1 second ($FEV_1$)) and forced vital capacity when combined with different classes of inhaled bronchodilators (long-acting muscarinic antagonists and $\beta_2$-agonists). In a Cochrane review across 20 randomised controlled trials involving patients with variable COPD severity (Ram et al. 2002), theophylline conferred small improvements in $FEV_1$ (100 mL) and arterial blood gas tensions compared to placebo (with little or no benefit on exercise tolerance and quality of life), although the incidence of nausea was significantly higher with active drug. It is important to note that few recent studies have investigated effects of theophylline in patients taking new and more potent long-acting bronchodilators.

The slow onset of action of theophylline combined with the necessary dose titration to achieve suitable plasma levels means that benefit may not be observed for several weeks. As with most drugs in COPD, clinicians should discontinue it if a therapeutic trial is unsuccessful. Low doses of theophylline may still confer benefit, perhaps because of enhanced activity of histone deacetylase (and increased corticosteroid sensitivity in individuals who smoke) and suppression of inflammation.

## Adverse effects

One of the main limitations preventing more extensive prescribing of theophylline is its propensity to cause dose-dependent adverse effects (Box 8.1), in addition to numerous patient characteristics and drugs that alter its half-life (Box 8.2).

---

Box 8.1 **Adverse effects of theophylline.**

- Tachycardia
- Cardiac arrhythmias
- Palpitation
- Nausea and vomiting
- Abdominal pain
- Gastric irritation
- Diarrhoea
- Headache
- Irritability and insomnia
- Seizures
- Hypokalaemia

---

Box 8.2 **Drugs and patient characteristics which alter plasma theophylline concentration.**

- Causes of increased plasma theophylline levels (i.e. reduced plasma clearance)
  - Heart failure
  - Liver cirrhosis
  - Advanced age
  - Ciprofloxacin
  - Erythromycin
  - Clarithromycin
  - Verapamil
  - Oestrogens
- Causes of reduced plasma theophylline levels (i.e. increased plasma clearance)
  - Cigarette smokers
  - Chronic alcoholism
  - Rifampicin
  - Phenytoin
  - Carbamazepine
  - Lithium
  - Sulfinpyrazone

---

The plasma concentration of theophylline should be checked when initially titrating the dose upwards, or when adding in a new drug that may alter its metabolism. Target levels between 10–20 mg/L (55–110 µM) reflect the 'bronchodilator window', whereas lower levels of 5–10 mg/mL are associated with anti-inflammatory and histone deacetylase activity. At theophylline concentrations greater than target levels, the frequency of adverse effects tends to increase to an unacceptable extent, although it can also arise when plasma levels fall well within the desired range. Check levels (4–6 hours after dosing with a modified-release preparation) 5 days after starting treatment and at least 3 days following dose adjustment (and titrate accordingly). During an exacerbation, reduce the dose of theophylline by 50% if a macrolide (e.g. clarithromycin) or fluoroquinolone (e.g. ciprofloxacin) is prescribed.

## Phosphodiesterase inhibitors

A group of more selective PDE inhibitors (PDE4 inhibitors) have been developed in an attempt to confer benefit with fewer adverse effects than theophylline (Calverley et al. 2009). The most clinically advanced drugs of this class are roflumilast and cilomolast. They act mainly as anti-inflammatory agents to reduce exacerbations but also have small bronchodilator effects. There are no head-to-head studies comparing theophylline and PDE4 inhibitors.

In a Cochrane review involving approximately 20 000 patients with COPD (Chong et al. 2013), studies involving treatment with a PDE4 inhibitor for at least 6 weeks were analysed. Treatment with a PDE4 inhibitor was associated with a significant although small (46 mL) improvement in $FEV_1$ versus placebo, plus benefits in quality of life and reduction in exacerbations. However, those receiving active treatment experienced more adverse events, such as gastrointestinal symptoms, headache, insomnia, weight loss and depression. The optimum place of PDE4 inhibitors in COPD management therefore remains to be defined, especially as it is uncertain if they confer any clinically meaningful benefit in patients taking maximal inhaled treatment. However, recent international guidelines have suggested that a PDE4 inhibitor is considered in patients with $FEV_1 < 50\%$ predicted, especially those with chronic bronchitis taking maximal inhaled therapy.

## Oral corticosteroids

Although COPD is associated with an abnormal local and systemic inflammatory response, oral corticosteroids have a limited role in the management of stable disease (Walters et al. 2005). Despite their long-term use in some patients (especially those with more advanced airflow obstruction and frequent exacerbations), typically prednisolone, there is little or no evidence supporting this practice, while discontinuation of long-term systemic corticosteroids has not been shown to cause a significant increase in COPD exacerbations. Long-term oral corticosteroids have unwanted effects on skeletal muscle and diaphragmatic function, which may well compound existing respiratory muscle weakness along with a multitude of other short-, medium- and long-term multisystem adverse effects. Therefore, avoid long-term corticosteroid use wherever possible (Figures 8.3, 8.4, 8.5).

In clinical practice, there are some severely symptomatic patients with advanced airflow obstruction in whom it is difficult to discontinue corticosteroids following an exacerbation, although this may in part be due to mood-enhancing effects. In situations where withdrawal is impossible, the lowest possible dose (such as 5 mg/day of prednisolone) may be considered.

### Prevention of corticosteroid-associated adverse effects

Before starting oral corticosteroids, patients should know the dose of drug to be taken, its anticipated duration and some of the potential adverse effects. Inform individuals receiving long-term oral corticosteroids that they should not be stopped suddenly and a slow reduction in dose is usually necessary prior to discontinuation. Immediate withdrawal after prolonged administration may lead to

acute adrenal insufficiency and even death. Therefore, issue all patients receiving oral corticosteroids with a treatment card alerting others (which also serves as a reminder to themselves) about the problems associated with abrupt discontinuation (Figure 8.6). Courses of oral corticosteroids which last less than 3 weeks (e.g. given to treat an exacerbation of COPD) do not generally need to be tapered before stopping.

The risk of corticosteroid-induced osteoporosis is related to cumulative dose. This implies that in addition to individuals receiving maintenance prednisolone, those requiring frequent courses may experience long-term complications. Patients using at least 7.5 mg/day of prednisolone (or equivalent) for 3 months are at heightened risk of adverse effects, along with those over the age of 65 years. The greatest rate of bone loss occurs within the first year of use, which means that early steps to prevent osteoporosis should be considered.

Bisphosphonates impair osteoclast function and therefore reduce bone turnover. This class of drug is useful in both the prevention and treatment of corticosteroid-related osteoporosis. Dual-energy X-ray absorptiometry (DXA) scans can facilitate early identification of patients at risk of corticosteroid-associated adverse effects. They also highlight which patients should commence a weekly bisphosphonate (e.g. risedronate or alendronate). Those over the age of 65 years, with or without a low trauma/fragility fracture, should commence oral bisphosphonate therapy

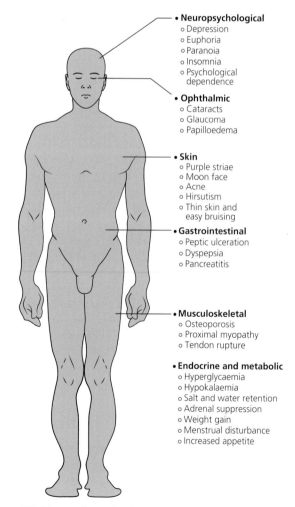

- **Neuropsychological**
  o Depression
  o Euphoria
  o Paranoia
  o Insomnia
  o Psychological dependence
- **Ophthalmic**
  o Cataracts
  o Glaucoma
  o Papilloedema
- **Skin**
  o Purple striae
  o Moon face
  o Acne
  o Hirsutism
  o Thin skin and easy bruising
- **Gastrointestinal**
  o Peptic ulceration
  o Dyspepsia
  o Pancreatitis
- **Musculoskeletal**
  o Osteoporosis
  o Proximal myopathy
  o Tendon rupture
- **Endocrine and metabolic**
  o Hyperglycaemia
  o Hypokalaemia
  o Salt and water retention
  o Adrenal suppression
  o Weight gain
  o Menstrual disturbance
  o Increased appetite

**Figure 8.3** Adverse effects of oral corticosteroids.

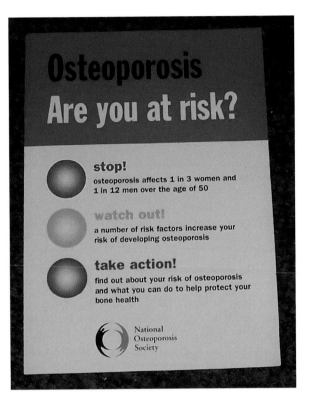

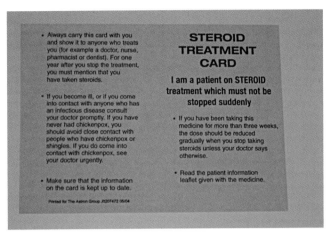

**Figure 8.6** All patients receiving oral corticosteroids should carry a treatment card at all times.

**Figure 8.4** Patients receiving frequent courses of, or maintained on, long-term oral corticosteroids should be aware of the risks of osteoporosis. Such patients should ensure an adequate intake of dietary calcium and be encouraged to exercise. Postmenopausal women should consider using hormone replacement therapy.

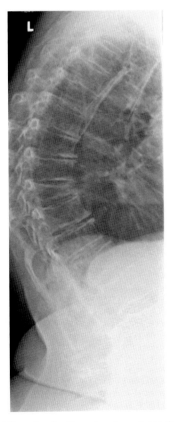

**Figure 8.5** Lateral thoracic spine X-ray showing osteopenia and an osteoporotic vertebral collapse in a patient using long-term oral corticosteroids; this elderly patient was not using a bisphosphonate.

at the onset of corticosteroid therapy and be referred, where possible, for DXA scanning. Those less than 65 years should be referred for DXA scanning at the time of commencing oral corticosteroids.

## Mucolytics

As increased oxidative stress and inflammation play a role in the pathogenesis of COPD, drugs with antioxidant and anti-inflammatory properties, such as N-acetylcysteine which can also act as a mucolytic, have been studied. However, studies evaluating mucolytics have shown inconsistent effects, while methodological drawbacks have been identified.

In one study (Decramer et al. 2005), 523 patients with COPD were randomised to receive N-acetylcysteine or placebo. After 3 years, no differences in exacerbations were identified, but in a smaller study, the frequency of exacerbations with N-acetylcysteine versus placebo was reduced (Tse et al. 2013). In a further study (Zheng et al. 2014), 1006 Chinese patients with moderate-to-severe COPD were randomised to receive N-acetylcysteine 600 mg twice daily or placebo. After 1 year, there were significantly fewer exacerbations with active treatment versus placebo (497 versus 641 respectively). However, many patients, especially in the latter two studies, were not using maximal inhaled treatment, while other drawbacks with these studies have been identified suggesting that outcomes may not be representative of the COPD population as a whole. In a Cochrane review involving over 9000 patients with COPD (or chronic bronchitis) (Poole et al. 2015), it was felt that a regular mucolytic may be associated with a small reduction in exacerbations and a small improvement in quality of life. In the same study, beneficial effects were less marked than those demonstrated in earlier studies.

Carbocisteine is the most commonly prescribed mucolytic in the UK and is generally well tolerated. It should be used with caution in those with peptic ulceration as it may disrupt the gastric mucosal barrier. A mucolytic may be considered in patients with cough productive of sputum in an attempt to help expectorate by reducing sputum viscosity, especially if they experience frequent exacerbations. This class of drug should not be routinely used unless data emerge in the future as to which patients are most likely to derive benefit, and that such benefit is considered to be worthwhile. Erdosteine is another mucolytic which can be considered for up to 10 days during an acute exacerbation of COPD.

## Long-term antibiotics

In recent years, regular long-term antibiotics, typically macrolides, have been studied for the prophylaxis of exacerbations in some patients with COPD (Seemungal et al. 2008). In addition to antimicrobial effects, macrolides also exhibit immunomodulatory and anti-inflammatory properties. In a randomised controlled study (Albert et al. 2011), 1142 patients received 250 mg/daily of azithromycin or placebo (in addition to their usual drugs for COPD). After 1 year, those using azithromycin experienced a 17% reduction in exacerbations, although macrolide resistance was significantly higher with active treatment versus placebo (81% versus 41% respectively). In a Cochrane review of seven studies involving >3000 patients with COPD (Herath and Poole 2013), continuous prophylactic macrolides reduced exacerbations, although a clinically meaningful effect on quality of life was not achieved, with no change in lung function, frequency of hospital admissions or mortality.

Given concerns related to potential adverse effects such as antibiotic resistance, hearing disturbance, gastrointestinal effects, prolongation of the QTc interval (especially in patients at risk of cardiac arrhythmias), widespread continuous macrolide treatment to prevent exacerbations of COPD is not advocated. However, some clinicians may consider treatment with a macrolide in some individuals with more advanced disease who experience frequent exacerbations (despite good adherence to maximal inhaled treatment and exclusion of correctable trigger factors). In such patients, it is reasonable to consider that, if continuous macrolides are prescribed, it should be done on a trial basis, with a low threshold for discontinuation if no beneficial effect is found after a predefined period (perhaps over at least 3–6 months).

## β-Blockers

Since cigarette smoking is one of the main risk factors in the aetiology of cardiovascular diseases and COPD, many patients develop both conditions. Although historical concerns exist about β-blockers prescribed for cardiovascular diseases worsening the degree of airflow obstruction in COPD (especially in those with severe airflow obstruction), studies have generally indicated this fear to be unfounded. Moreover, an increasing body of evidence has accumulated indicating that they may be associated with reductions in mortality and exacerbation frequency, and improved survival when continued during an exacerbation of COPD (Figure 8.7) (Ekstrom et al. 2013; Short et al. 2011; van Gestel et al. 2008).

In one study of over 3000 patients (mean $FEV_1$ around 50% and of whom almost a third were receiving oxygen) over 2 years (Bhatt et al. 2016), β-blockers were associated with a significant reduction in exacerbations (irrespective of severity of airflow obstruction), with the benefit persisting after adjustment for underlying cardiovascular disease. Since other cardiac drugs were not associated with

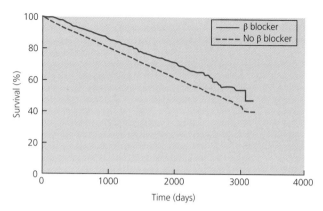

**Figure 8.7** Kaplan–Meier estimate of probability of survival among patients with COPD by use of β-blockers. Figure reproduced with permission from Short et al. [13].

a reduction in exacerbations, the implication was that the benefit of β-blockers was likely to be a class effect. In a meta-analysis of 15 retrospective studies of 21 596 patients with COPD, the pooled estimate for reduction in overall mortality conferred by β-blockers was 28%, and 38% for exacerbations (Du et al. 2014). In keeping with current guidelines, the prescription of a $\beta_1$-selective blocker such as bisoprolol or nebovolol should not be precluded in patients who have COPD plus left ventricular dysfunction or coronary artery disease who are likely to derive benefit (McMurray et al. 2012), although routine prescription in patients with COPD alone (without cardiovascular disease) is not advocated. The dose should be slowly titrated to help ensure both cardiac and pulmonary tolerability. Non-selective drugs such as carvedilol should be avoided in COPD as they increase the propensity for bronchoconstriction (Dungen et al. 2011; Jabbour et al. 2010).

## Other drugs

Cough is frequently a troublesome symptom in many patients, although it may, in fact, be advantageous, especially in patients who produce copious amounts of sputum. Antitussives are not known to provide any benefit in COPD, other than perhaps short-term symptomatic control of cough; their regular use should be discouraged. Other drugs such as statins and vitamin D have been studied in COPD, but no consistent beneficial effects have been identified.

In patients with cor pulmonale, there is no evidence that drugs such as angiotensin-converting enzyme inhibitors, angiotensin II receptor antagonists, digoxin, β-blockers or calcium channel blockers are of benefit. If measures such as leg elevation and compression stockings and, where appropriate, long-term oxygen therapy fail to control symptomatic peripheral oedema, low-dose diuretics can be tried. In such circumstances, monitor renal function carefully.

## Acknowledgment

The authors would like to thank Dr Rosemary Hollick, Department of Rheumatology, Aberdeen Royal Infirmary for commenting on parts of this chapter.

# References

Albert RK, Connett J, Bailey WC et al. Azithromycin for prevention of exacerbations of COPD. *New England Journal of Medicine* 2011; **365**: 689–698.

Barnes PJ. Theophylline: new perspectives for an old drug. *American Journal of Respiratory and Critical Care Medicine* 2003; **167**: 813–818.

Bhatt SP, Wells JM, Kinney GL et al. Beta-blockers are associated with a reduction in COPD exacerbations. *Thorax* 2016; **71**: 8–14.

Calverley PM, Rabe KF, Goehring UM, Kristiansen S, Fabbri LM, Martinez FJ. Roflumilast in symptomatic chronic obstructive pulmonary disease: two randomised clinical trials. *Lancet* 2009; **374**: 685–694.

Chong J, Leung B, Poole P. Phosphodiesterase 4 inhibitors for chronic obstructive pulmonary disease. *Cochrane Database of Systematic Reviews* 2013; **11**: CD002309.

Decramer M, Rutten-van Molken M, Dekhuijzen PN et al. Effects of N-acetylcysteine on outcomes in chronic obstructive pulmonary disease (Bronchitis Randomized on NAC Cost-Utility Study, BRONCUS): a randomised placebo-controlled trial. *Lancet* 2005; **365**: 1552–1560.

Du Q, Sun Y, Ding N, Lu L, Chen Y. Beta-blockers reduced the risk of mortality and exacerbation in patients with COPD: a meta-analysis of observational studies. *PLoS One* 2014; **9**: e113048.

Dungen HD, Apostolovic S, Inkrot S et al. Titration to target dose of bisoprolol vs. carvedilol in elderly patients with heart failure: the CIBIS-ELD trial. *European Journal of Heart Failure* 2011; **13**: 670–680.

Ekstrom MP, Hermansson AB, Strom KE. Effects of cardiovascular drugs on mortality in severe chronic obstructive pulmonary disease. *American Journal of Respiratory and Critical Care Medicine* 2013; **187**: 715–720.

Herath SC, Poole P. Prophylactic antibiotic therapy for chronic obstructive pulmonary disease (COPD). *Cochrane Database of Systematic Reviews* 2013; **11**: CD009764.

Jabbour A, Macdonald PS, Keogh AM et al. Differences between beta-blockers in patients with chronic heart failure and chronic obstructive pulmonary disease: a randomized crossover trial. *Journal of the American College of Cardiology* 2010; **55**: 1780–1787.

McMurray JJ, Adamopoulos S, Anker SD et al. ESC guidelines for the diagnosis and treatment of acute and chronic heart failure 2012: the Task Force for the Diagnosis and Treatment of Acute and Chronic Heart Failure 2012 of the European Society of Cardiology. Developed in collaboration with the Heart Failure Association (HFA) of the ESC. *European Journal of Heart Failure* 2012; **14**: 803–869.

Poole P, Chong J, Cates CJ. Mucolytic agents versus placebo for chronic bronchitis or chronic obstructive pulmonary disease. *Cochrane Database of Systematic Reviews* 2015; **7**: CD001287.

Ram FS, Jones PW, Castro AA et al. Oral theophylline for chronic obstructive pulmonary disease. *Cochrane Database of Systematic Reviews* 2002; **4**: CD003902.

Seemungal TA, Wilkinson TM, Hurst JR, Perera WR, Sapsford RJ, Wedzicha JA. Long-term erythromycin therapy is associated with decreased chronic obstructive pulmonary disease exacerbations. *American Journal of Respiratory and Critical Care Medicine* 2008; **178**: 1139–147.

Short PM, Lipworth SI, Elder DH, Schembri S, Lipworth BJ. Effect of beta blockers in treatment of chronic obstructive pulmonary disease: a retrospective cohort study. *BMJ* 2011; **342**: d2549.

Tse HN, Raiteri L, Wong KY et al. High-dose N-acetylcysteine in stable COPD: the 1-year, double-blind, randomized, placebo-controlled HIACE study. *Chest* 2013; **144**: 106–118.

Van Gestel YR, Hoeks SE, Sin DD et al. Impact of cardioselective beta-blockers on mortality in patients with chronic obstructive pulmonary disease and atherosclerosis. *American Journal of Respiratory and Critical Care Medicine* 2008; **178**: 695–700.

Walters JA, Walters EH, Wood-Baker R. Oral corticosteroids for stable chronic obstructive pulmonary disease. *Cochrane Database of Systematic Reviews* 2005; **3**: CD005374.

Zheng JP, Wen FQ, Bai CX et al. Twice daily N-acetylcysteine 600 mg for exacerbations of chronic obstructive pulmonary disease (PANTHEON): a randomised, double-blind placebo-controlled trial. *Lancet Respiratory Medicine* 2014; **2**: 187–194.

# CHAPTER 9

# Drug Delivery Devices

*Morag Reilly[1], Graham Douglas[2] and Graeme P. Currie[2]*

[1] Aberdeen City Health and Social Care Community Partnership, Aberdeen, UK
[2] Aberdeen Royal Infirmary, Aberdeen, UK

---

## OVERVIEW

- Initial demonstration and regular assessment of inhaler technique are often neglected in the overall care of patients with chronic obstructive pulmonary disease.

- Give patients specific instructions on use of the particular inhaler and ensure they can use it with confidence.

- Assess inhaler technique at every available opportunity as technique declines over time.

- The two main types of inhaler are aerosol based (which require slow inhalation) and dry powder inhalers (which require fast inhalation).

- A pressurised metered dose inhaler (pMDI) should ideally be used with a compatible spacer.

- Dry powder inhalers (DPIs) reduce the need for co-ordination and are easier to use than pMDIs.

- If a patient is unable to use a particular device, consider an alternative.

- Only consider delivering bronchodilators by nebuliser in those with persistent severe symptoms and advanced airflow obstruction (who demonstrate subjective and/or objective benefit), and in those unable to use inhalers correctly.

---

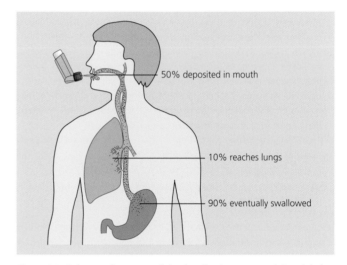

**Figure 9.1** Only a small amount of the drug leaving a metered dose inhaler reaches the lungs.

Drugs have been administered by inhalation for thousands of years. For example, between 2000 and 1500 BC in Egypt and India, herbal preparations were burned and the vapours inhaled. Over subsequent years, a variety of medicinal and non-medicinal substances were inhaled as treatments for breathlessness, and eventually a primitive nebuliser was developed in the mid-1800s. In 1929, the potential benefits of inhaled adrenaline were reported for patients with obstructive lung disorders and pressurised metered dose inhalers (pMDIs) were introduced in the 1950s.

Most drugs used in chronic obstructive pulmonary disease (COPD) are inhaled through the mouth using hand-held devices. This makes intuitive sense as this route of delivery means that drugs are delivered topically to the airways. Unfortunately, even with optimal inhaler technique, only a small proportion of inhaled drug reaches the lungs, as a considerable amount is deposited in the mouth, throat and vocal

cords and subsequently swallowed (Figure 9.1). Trying to ensure the best possible inhaler technique is paramount as evidence suggests that as many as 50% of patients fail to correctly use their inhaler sufficiently well to derive benefit from the prescribed drug. Nevertheless, if inhalers are used correctly, all types of device generally have similar clinical efficacy. No 'perfect' inhaler exists but characteristics of the optimum inhaler device are shown in Box 9.1.

---

Box 9.1 **Attributes of the 'perfect' inhaler.**

- Ease of use during an acute episode of breathlessness
- Ease of use as maintenance treatment
- As few steps as possible to operate
- Quick delivery of drug
- Portable and lightweight
- Same type of inhaler for different drugs
- Ease of co-ordinating inhalation manoeuvre

---

- Confirmation of dose delivery
- A dose counter to reflect how many inhalations remain
- Inexpensive
- Harmless to the environment
- Little or no maintenance or cleaning required
- Inhaler durability
- No special storage requirements once opened

---

Box 9.2 **Practical aids to teaching inhaler technique.**

- Ensure it is delivered by a professional trained in correct inhaler technique
- Decide whether to use a dry powder inhaler or pMDI
- Try to have a first- and second-line choice for both DPI or pMDI
- Try to use the same type of inhaler (i.e. DPI or pMDI) for additional drugs
- Talk through how to use the inhaler with the patient
- Demonstrate how to use the device (usually with a placebo)
- Ask for patient feedback and check if they understand how to use the device
- Answer any queries – the demonstration might need to be repeated
- Ask the patient to practically demonstrate the technique to you (using a placebo)
- Give verbal feedback and highlight any errors
- Repeat the process until satisfactory technique is observed
- Consider switching device or addition of a spacer for a pMDI if unable to optimise patient inhaler technique

## Choosing the correct inhaler

An increasingly bewildering array of inhaler devices is now available and problems often arise for both the health care provider and patient as to which type is most suitable. Many advantages and disadvantages of different inhaler types exist.

The two main types of inhaler are:
- pressurised metered dose inhalers (pMDIs): these are aerosol based and mixed with a pressurised hydrofluoroalkane (HFA) propellant to deliver drug to the lungs; some newer generation aerosol inhalers use a suspension and are propellant free
- dry powder inhalers (DPIs): these require the patient's own inspiratory effort to deliver drug to the lungs.

Optimal inhaler technique for each type is markedly different.
- pMDIs provide optimal lung deposition with a *slow* inhalation; full inhalation should take 5–10 seconds.
- DPIs require higher inspiratory flow rates and inhalation should therefore be *fast* but also for as long as possible.

To ensure the device selected is suitable for the patients' individual needs, consider the most appropriate inhaler device group (i.e. pMDI or DPI) and not just the drug required. Keep in mind the patient's age, as increased age is often associated with reduced manual dexterity and visual acuity, while learning and retaining new information may be problematic for some.

As COPD progresses, a greater number of inhaled drugs are required which can result in the need for more inhaler devices (with different techniques). This may confuse patients and hinder optimal inhaler technique, lung deposition and drug efficacy. Wherever possible, use the same inhaler device to deliver different drugs, but if not possible, try to be consistent between the use of aerosol-based inhalers or DPIs. Combination inhalers containing two drugs, e.g. inhaled corticosteroid and long-acting $\beta_2$-agonist, may be appropriate as COPD progresses.

When prescribing an inhaler, the overriding principles are:
- ability of the patient to use the device correctly and consistently
- adequate instruction given by someone skilled in doing so
- keeping the use of different devices to a minimum
- patient preference
- ease of use.

## Errors in patient inhaler technique

Studies demonstrate that poor inhaler technique is common. Incorrect inhaler technique is more likely with:
- increased age
- lower levels of education
- low levels of instruction on inhaler technique
- use of multiple different inhaler devices
- multiple steps required to operate the inhaler.

Some errors are common to both pMDIs and DPIs, while others are device specific. The most common errors in technique, depending on type of device, are shown in Table 9.1.

## Teaching and checking patient inhaler technique

It is important that assessment and correction of inhaler technique are carried out at every available opportunity (Box 9.2). This is because, over time, patients often become less able to use their inhaler correctly. Training methods include:
- verbal instruction
- written instruction
- practical demonstration
- interactive computer programs
- audiovisual demonstration.

Additional information a patient needs to know about their inhaler device includes:

Table 9.1  Common errors with pMDIs and DPIs.

| Error | pMDI | DPI |
| --- | --- | --- |
| Failure to shake the device before use | √ | n/a |
| Failure to exhale to residual volume before inhalation | √ | √ |
| Exhaling into mouthpiece before use | √ | √ |
| Failure to co-ordinate actuation and inhalation | √ | n/a |
| Inhalation too fast | √ | n/a |
| Inhalation too slow | n/a | √ |
| Inadequate breath hold after inspiration | √ | √ |
| Multiple actuations of device during single inspiration | √ | n/a |
| Exhaling into mouthpiece after use | √ | √ |
| Holding device incorrectly | √ | √ |
| Priming device incorrectly | n/a | √ |

- whether it needs priming before use for the first time (if so, how this is performed)
- the number of doses the inhaler contains
- how long it should last
- how to determine when the device is empty
- how to clean the device
- who to speak to if problems arise (and how to contact them).

## Different types of inhalers

Many different types of inhaler devices are available, all of which have their own particular advantages, disadvantages and character-istics (Tables 9.2, 9.3).

### Metered dose inhaler

The most widely available inhaler device is the pMDI (Figure 9.2). Since the Montreal protocol in January 1989, all pMDIs are required to be chlorofluorocarbon (CFC) propellant free. HFA propellants are now used which deliver the aerosol plume at a lower force, and feel and taste very different from traditional CFC pMDIs. When the content of the inhaler is released, it undergoes volume expansion and forms a mixture of gas and liquid before being discharged as a jet through the orifice of the actuator. Following aerosolisation and dispersion into multiple droplets, and during propulsion of these droplets from the actuator, the drug particles within the droplets become progressively concentrated. This is due to rapid evapora-tion of the volatile propellant components.

pMDIs deliver short-acting $\beta_2$-agonist (SABA) monotherapy, long-acting $\beta_2$-agonist (LABA) monotherapy, inhaled corticoster-oid (ICS) monotherapy, or a LABA and ICS in combination (Box 9.3). Patients often have difficulty using pMDIs, particularly co-ordinating actuation of the device with adequate inspiratory effort. Moreover, radiolabelled studies have shown that only around 10% of the emitted drug reaches the lungs, even with good technique.

---

**Box 9.3 How to use a pMDI.**

- Remove the mouthpiece cover (if there is one) and shake the inhaler
- Hold the inhaler upright with the thumb on the base and first finger on top of the canister
- Exhale fully (taking care not to breathe into the pMDI)
- Place lips (and teeth) firmly around the mouthpiece to ensure a good seal (ensure the tongue does not obstruct the mouthpiece)
- Breathe in slowly and deeply; when starting to inhale, depress the canister to release a dose of drug
- Continue to breathe in slowly and deeply for as long as possible, at least 5 seconds
- Remove the inhaler from the mouth
- Hold breath for up to 10 seconds or for as long as comfortable
- Exhale normally
- Repeat after 30 seconds if a second dose is required
- Wipe the mouthpiece clean and replace mouthpiece cover

---

**Table 9.2** Advantages and disadvantages of different types of inhaler devices.

| Type of inhaler | Advantages | Disadvantages |
|---|---|---|
| Metered dose inhaler (pMDI) | • Portable<br>• Inexpensive<br>• Short treatment time<br>• Contain high numbers of doses | • Actuation and inhalation co-ordination required<br>• High potential for poor technique<br>• Sometimes no dose counter |
| Metered dose inhaler with spacer | • More effective drug delivery<br>• Reduced oropharyngeal drug deposition<br>• Useful in emergency situations<br>• Most patients manage to use a pMDI and spacer when unable to use other devices | • Less portable<br>• Maintenance required to overcome electrostatic charges<br>• Sometimes no dose counter<br>• Due to licence, some spacers are only for use with specific brands of pMDI |
| Dry powder inhaler (DPI):<br>Turbohaler, Accuhaler, Handihaler, Ellipta, Genuair, Breezhaler, Spiromax, Nexthaler | • No actuation/inhalation co-ordination necessary<br>• Portable<br>• Usually have a dose counter<br>• Usually have very little taste<br>• Spacer unnecessary<br>• Short treatment time | • Adequate inspiratory flow required<br>• Often more expensive than pMDIs<br>• No propellant<br>• Carrier often lactose (ask if an intolerance is present)<br>• Should not be stored in damp environments |
| Breath-activated metered dose inhaler:<br>Easibreathe and Autohaler | • No actuation/inhalation co-ordination necessary<br>• Portable<br>• Short treatment time | • Adequate inspiratory flow required |
| Slow mist inhaler (Respimat) | • Portable<br>• Effective with smaller drug doses | • No propellant<br>• Actuation and inhalation co-ordination required (less than for pMDI) |
| Nebuliser | • Tidal breathing adequate<br>• Easy to use<br>• Patient preference | • Less portable, noisy and indiscreet<br>• Expensive and maintenance required<br>• Unpredictable lung deposition<br>• Variable performance<br>• Drug wastage<br>• Long drug delivery time<br>• Need for a power source |

**Table 9.3** Features of different inhaler devices available for COPD patients.

| Device name | Inhaler type | Class of drugs delivered in COPD | Priming before 1st use required | Initial shake required | Characteristics of inhalation | Length of breath hold required | Capsule to be inserted | Dose counter | How to store/use by | Special notes |
|---|---|---|---|---|---|---|---|---|---|---|
| pMDI | pMDI | SABA LABA ICS/LABA | Yes | Yes | Slow and long | 10 sec | No | Sometimes | Do not store above 25°C | Spacer and/or Haleraid can be added |
| Easibreathe | Breath-actuated pMDI | SABA | No | Yes | Slow and long | 10 sec | No | No | Do not store above 25°C | None |
| Autohaler | Breath-actuated pMDI | SABA | Yes | Yes | Slow and long | 10 sec | No | No | Store below 30°C | None |
| Respimat | Soft mist | LAMA LAMA/LABA | Yes | No | Slow and long | 10 sec | No | Yes | Use within 3 months of first use | None |
| Accuhaler (Diskus) | DPI | SABA LABA ICS/LABA | No | No | Fast and long | 10 sec | No | Yes | Do not store above 30°C | Contains lactose |
| Turbohaler | DPI | SABA LABA ICS/LABA | Yes | No | Fast and long | 10 sec | No | Yes | Do not store above 30°C | Contains lactose |
| Handihaler | DPI | LAMA | No | No | Fast and long | 10 secs | Yes | N/A | Store sealed capsules between 20–25°C | Contains lactose |
| Breezhaler | DPI | LABA LAMA LABA/LAMA | No | No | Fast and long | 10 sec | Yes | N/A | Do not store above 30°C. Dispose of inhaler after 30 days of use | Contains lactose |
| Ellipta | DPI | LAMA LAMA/LABA ICS/LAMA | No | No | Fast and long | 3–4 sec | No | Yes | Do not store above 25°C. Use within 6 weeks of opening | Contains lactose |
| Genuair | DPI | LAMA LAMA/LABA | No | No | Fast and long | As long as comfortable | No | Yes Locks when empty | Use within 60 days of opening | Contains lactose |
| Nexthaler | DPI | ICS/LABA | No | No | Fast and long | 10 sec | No | Yes | Do not store above 25°C once opened. Use within 6 months of opening | Contains lactose |
| Spiromax | DPI | ICS/LABA | No | No | Fast and long | 10 sec | No | Yes | Do not store above 25°C. Use within 6 months of opening | Contains lactose |

DPI, dry powder inhaler; ICS, inhaled corticosteroid; LABA, long-acting β₂-agonist; LAMA, long-acting muscarinic antagonist; pMDI, pressurised metered dose inhaler; SABA, short-acting β₂-agonist.

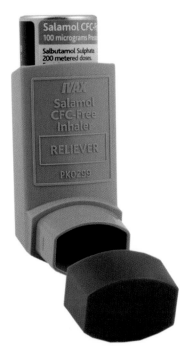

**Figure 9.2** A pressurised metered dose inhaler.

Most new pMDIs require test firing before use for the first time. This usually involves shaking the inhaler and then releasing 2-4 puffs from the inhaler into the air. Instructions vary between manufacturers and should be checked individually. Test firing is also usually advised if the pMDI has not been used for a few days/weeks.

Many pMDIs contain a small amount of ethanol (alcohol) and may therefore not be suitable for some patients. To help establish when the device is empty, some pMDIs include a dose counter. This usually counts backwards to zero. If a pMDI does not have a dose counter, a practical way to determine when it is empty is to write the date the inhaler was started on the device and manually record the number of doses taken.

### Haleraid

Haleraid is a hinged plastic device with a handle that fits over some types of pMDI (Figure 9.3). It provides extra leverage for the patient; when the handle is squeezed, the inhaler is activated. It is designed to assist patients who have difficulty in pressing down on the pMDI canister due to problems with manual strength or dexterity.

### Metered dose inhaler plus spacer

A spacer device is a valved chamber (some can have a mask) that can be attached to a pMDI to help avoid problems in co-ordinating the timing of actuation and inhalation (Figure 9.4). It also overcomes the 'cold freon' effect whereby the cold blast of propellant reaching the oropharynx results in cessation of inhalation or inhalation through the nose (usually less of a problem in inhalers using HFA compared to older CFC propellants). If used correctly, a pMDI with spacer is at least as effective for delivery of inhaled drugs as any other device. Different manufacturers make different sizes of spacers and inhalers and may require matching by brand.

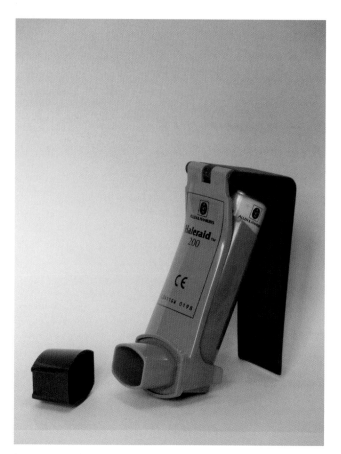

**Figure 9.3** A Haleraid.

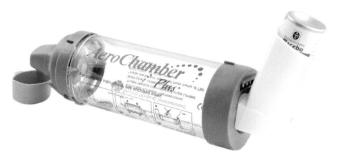

**Figure 9.4** A metered dose inhaler with spacer.

Aerosol drug particles delivered into a spacer may adhere to the chamber walls by electrostatic attraction. Washing the spacer can reduce this problem. Spacers should generally be cleaned at least once a month using lukewarm water with mild liquid detergent and left to drip dry. They should be replaced every 6–12 months, depending on the manufacturer's recommendations.

Some patients develop oropharyngeal candidiasis and complain of an alteration in the voice quality (dysphonia) when using an inhaler without a spacer to deliver inhaled corticosteroids (Figure 9.5). The risk of developing these problems can be minimised by gargling with water and mouth rinsing after inhaler use or by using a spacer device with a pMDI to reduce upper airway drug deposition.

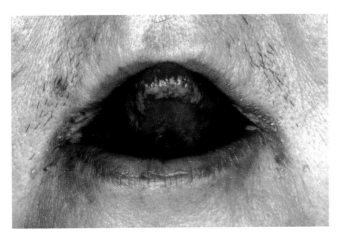

**Figure 9.5** Oropharyngeal candidiasis in a patient incorrectly using a pMDI containing high-dose inhaled corticosteroids.

There are two ways to use a pMDI and spacer (Box 9.4). Both are equally as effective; which is used depends on patient ability, preference and circumstance of use.

---

Box 9.4 **Two ways to use a pMDI and spacer.**

**Single breath technique**
- Remove the protective cap from the spacer and inhaler
- Ensure the spacer is empty
- Check the inhaler fits tightly into the end of the spacer
- Briskly shake the whole unit a few times
- Exhale fully (away from the spacer and inhaler)
- Place teeth and lips around the mouthpiece (ensure tongue does not obstruct the mouthpiece)
- Press the inhaler once*
- With minimum delay, breathe inwards fully, slowly and deeply (some spacers create a whistling noise if technique is incorrect, indicating inhalation is too fast)
- Hold breath for up to 10 seconds or as long as is comfortable
- Remove spacer from the mouth
- Wait 30 seconds before repeating these steps if a second dose is required
- Wipe the mouthpiece clean

**Tidal breathing technique**
- Perform steps above as for single breath technique to*
- With minimum delay, breathe inwards fully, slowly and deeply then slowly exhale though the mouth into the spacer
- Continue to inhale and exhale as described for 4–5 breaths (some spacers create a whistling noise if technique is incorrect, indicating inhalation is too fast)
- Remove spacer from the mouth
- Wait 30 seconds before repeating these steps if a second dose is required
- Wipe the mouthpiece clean

---

## Breath-activated pMDIs

These types of inhalers (Easibreathe and Autohaler) were developed to overcome problems of co-ordination associated with pMDIs. When a patient inhales through the trigger device, a mechanism

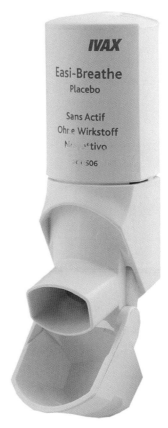

**Figure 9.6** An Easibreathe inhaler.

automatically 'fires' the breath-activated MDI with subsequent release of drug. This means that inhalation and actuation coincide.

*Easibreathe inhaler*
The Easibreathe inhaler (Figure 9.6) delivers SABA or ICS monotherapy. For optimal lung deposition, inhalation must be *slow and long*. There is no dose counter on an Easibreathe, and once empty it is no longer possible to 'feel' or 'hear' propellant being dispensed (Box 9.5).

---

Box 9.5 **How to use an Easibreathe inhaler.**

- Shake the inhaler
- Hold the inhaler upright
- Open the cap, covering the mouthpiece by folding it down
- Hold the Easibreathe away from the mouth and exhale fully (taking care not to breathe into the device)
- Place lips around the mouthpiece and ensure a good seal (take care not to block the air holes on top of the device)
- Breathe inwards slowly, deeply and fully (a click will be heard)
- Continue to inhale
- Hold breath for up to 10 seconds or as long as comfortable
- Remove the inhaler from the mouth and gently exhale
- Close the mouthpiece cap
- Repeat these steps if a second dose is required
- Wipe the mouthpiece clean and replace the cap

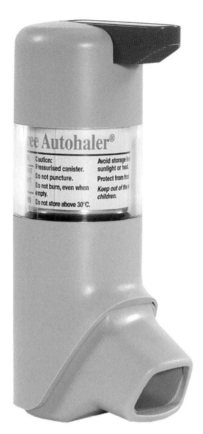

**Figure 9.7** An Autohaler.

*Autohaler*

Autohalers deliver SABA monotherapy (Figure 9.7). A new Autohaler requires preparing before it is used for the first time (Box 9.6). This process must also be performed if it has not been

---

**Box 9.6 How to prepare a new Autohaler.**

- Remove the cap covering the mouthpiece
- Shake the inhaler
- Hold the device upright and push the lever on top of the device up until it remains up
- Direct the mouthpiece of the inhaler away
- To release a puff from the inhaler, push the dose release slide on the bottom of the device in the direction indicated by the arrow
- To release the next dose, the lever on top of the inhaler needs to be returned to its down position and the steps above followed again; this process needs to be performed four times
- After the fourth puff, the lever must be returned to the 'down' position; having done so, the inhaler is ready for use

---

used for 2 weeks or more. There is no dose counter on an Autohaler, and once empty it is no longer possible to 'feel' or 'hear' any propellant being dispensed (Box 9.7).

**Box 9.7 How to use an Autohaler.**

- Remove the cap covering the mouthpiece
- Shake the inhaler
- Hold the device upright and push the lever on top of the device up until it remains up
- Continue to hold the device upright, taking care not to block the air vents at the bottom
- Hold the Autohaler away from the mouth and exhale fully (take care not to breathe into the device)
- Place lips around the mouthpiece and ensure a good seal
- Breathe inwards slowly, deeply and fully (a click will be heard)
- Continue to inhale
- Hold breath for up to 10 seconds or as long as comfortable
- Remove the inhaler from the mouth and gently exhale
- Ensure the lever on top of the device has returned to the 'down' position
- Repeat these steps if a second dose is required
- Wipe the mouthpiece clean and replace the cap

## Soft mist inhaler
### Respimat

Respimat is currently the only hand-held device delivering a slow-moving, soft mist (Figure 9.8). It is propellant free. A mist with low spray momentum is generated with small droplet size, resulting in a high level of drug deposition in the airways. The Respimat delivers LABA monotherapy or long acting muscarinic antagonist (LAMA) and LABA in combination.

A dose indicator on the side of the Respimat helps establish when the device is empty; a pointer starts at 60 and reduces to zero. When the pointer enters the red area of the scale, 14 inhalations remain. Once the dose indicator reaches zero the device automatically locks and cannot be used again.

A new Respimat requires loading and preparing before it is used for the first time (Box 9.8). If the Respimat has not been

---

**Box 9.8 Steps in loading and preparing a Respimat.**

**Step 1 Inserting the cartridge**
- With the cap of the device closed, press the safety catch while pulling off the clear base
- Take the cartridge out of the box and push the narrow end of the cartridge into the inhaler until it clicks
- Push the cartridge firmly against a solid surface, ensuring it connects with the end of the inhaler
- Replace the clear base; it does not need to be removed again

**Step 2 Preparing the Respimat for use**
- Hold the device upright with the cap closed
- Rotate the base in the direction of the black arrows on the label until it clicks
- Open the cap fully
- Point the inhaler towards the ground and press the dose release button
- Close the cap
- Repeat step 2 until a cloud is visible
- Repeat step 2 three more times
- The Respimat is now ready for use

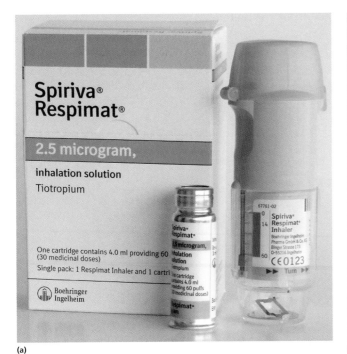

(a)

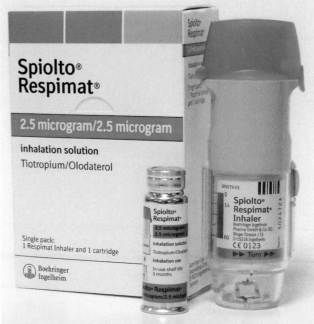

(b)

(c)

**Figure 9.8** Respimat soft mist inhalers.

for 7 days, one dose must be released towards the ground before use; if it has not been used for 21 days, step 2 must be repeated before use (Box 9.9).

---

Box 9.9 **How to use a Respimat.**

- Hold the inhaler upright with the cap closed
- Rotate the base in the direction of the black arrows until it clicks
- Open the cap fully
- Exhale fully (taking care not to breathe into the device)
- Close lips around the end of the mouthpiece to ensure a tight seal (taking care not to block air vents)

- Direct the inhaler towards the back of the throat
- Start to inhale slowly and deeply through the mouth and at the same time press the dose release button
- Continue to breathe in slowly for as long as possible
- Hold the breath for 10 seconds or for as long as possible
- Close the cap
- Repeat the process to obtain a second dose

---

## Dry powder inhalers

Dry powder inhalers used in COPD are all breath activated. This means that the inspiratory flow rate generated by the patient deaggregates the powder into smaller particles that are then dispersed within the lungs. The need for co-ordination is less than when using a pMDI without a spacer. Different DPIs require higher flow rates than pMDIs, meaning that a more forceful inhalation is required to deposit the drug within the lungs. This in turn may influence the type of DPI prescribed to patients, especially in those with more advanced airflow obstruction, hyperinflated lungs at rest and poor inspiratory reserve. As a general rule, however, if patients can perform spirometry, they usually have sufficient inspiratory flow to use most DPIs. Problems encountered with DPIs include failure to exhale to residual volume before use, exhaling into the mouthpiece, inadequate or no breath hold, failure to hold the device upright and failure to inhale with sufficient force.

## Accuhaler or Diskus

This device is termed Accuhaler in Australia and the UK, and Diskus in France and the US (Figure 9.9). These disk-shaped containers use a machined two-piece long foil ribbon with each unit dose held in small caplet-shaped depressions along the entire dose-count length. The Accuhaler delivers SABA monotherapy, LABA monotherapy, ICS monotherapy, or a LABA and ICS in combination (Box 9.10). The device also contains lactose and may be unsuitable for patients with intolerance. . To help establish when the device is empty, Accuhalers (like most DPIs) have a dose counter; this counts backwards to zero with the numbers 5 to 0 appearing in red to indicate that only a few doses remain.

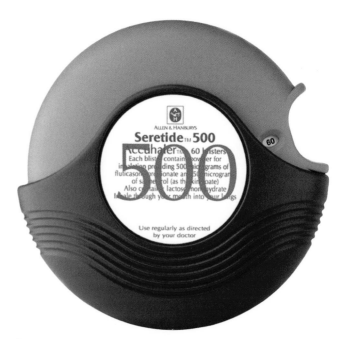

**Figure 9.9** An Accuhaler.

Box 9.10 **How to use an Accuhaler.**

- Open the device by holding the outer case in one hand and putting the thumb of the other hand on the grip
- Push the thumb grip away as far as it will go until a click is heard (this opens a small hole in the mouthpiece)
- Hold the device with the mouthpiece towards you
- Slide the small lever beside the thumb grip away as far as it will go (this results in a small click indicating the dose is ready for use)
- Hold the inhaler away from the mouth and exhale fully (taking care not to breathe into the Accuhaler)
- Put lips around the mouthpiece to ensure a tight seal
- Inhale quickly, deeply and fully
- Remove the inhaler from the mouth and hold breath for up to 10 seconds or as long as comfortable
- Exhale slowly
- Wipe the mouthpiece clean
- Close the device by sliding the thumb grip backwards until it clicks

## Turbohaler

A Turbohaler is a multidose dry powder device (Figure 9.10) that delivers SABA monotherapy, LABA monotherapy, ICS monotherapy, or ICS in combination with a LABA (Box 9.11).

The amount of drug inhaled using a Turbohaler is very small and a taste may not be apparent. This does not mean a dose has been missed, providing all steps in the process have been followed correctly. The device also contains lactose and may be unsuitable for patients with an intolerance.

To help establish when the device is empty, Turbohalers have a small indicator window on the side. A red mark appears at the top of the window when there are 20 doses left; when it reaches the bottom of the window, the Turbohaler is empty. If the Turbohaler

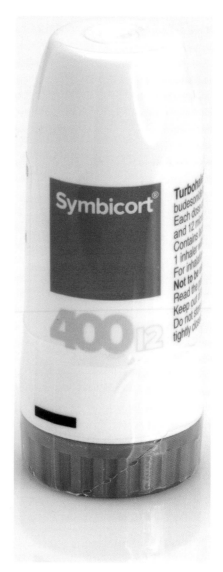

**Figure 9.10** A Turbohaler.

Box 9.11 **How to use a Turbohaler.**

- Unscrew the outer cover and remove it
- Hold the inhaler upright with the grip at the bottom
- Rotate the grip as far as it will go in one direction and then rotate it back as far as it will go in the other direction (which way it is turned first does not matter); a click should be heard indicating the Turbohaler is ready for use
- *If using a new Turbohaler for the first time, these initial steps will need to be repeated*
- Hold the Turbohaler away from the mouth and exhale fully (take care not to breathe into the Turbohaler)
- Place lips around the mouthpiece and ensure a good seal
- Inhale quickly, deeply and fully
- Hold breath for up to 10 seconds or as long as is comfortable
- Repeat these steps if a second dose is required
- Wipe the mouthpiece clean and replace the outer cover

contains an ICS and LABA combination, the indicator window will also include a numerical aid that will count down to zero. The sound heard when the Turbohaler is shaken is produced by a drying agent (and not the drug) and is therefore not an indicator of how much medicine remains.

## Handihaler

The Handihaler is a single-dose device that delivers LAMA tiotropium (Figure 9.11). It requires a capsule to be loaded into the device before use. Capsules should never be swallowed and only those designed for use in a Handihaler should be used (Box 9.12).

Box 9.12 **How to use a Handihaler.**

**Step 1 Load the inhaler**
- Open the outer lid by pulling it upwards
- Open the inner white mouthpiece by pulling it upwards; the centre chamber should now be visible
- Peel the foil from the blister to expose one capsule and remove it (only open the blister immediately before use)
- Place a capsule into the inner chamber in the centre of the Handihaler
- Close the mouthpiece firmly against the base until a click is heard

**Step 2 Pierce the capsule**
- Hold the Handihaler with the mouthpiece pointed upwards
- Press the button at the side of the inhaler *once* (this pierces the capsule) and release
- Do not press the button more than once or shake the inhaler

**Step 3 Inhale the drug**
- Hold the Handihaler away from the mouth and exhale fully (take care not to breathe into the device)
- Place lips around the mouthpiece and ensure a good seal
- Breathe inwards quickly, deeply and fully (a rattling sound should be heard)
- Hold breath for up to 10 seconds or as long as is comfortable
- Remove the inhaler from the mouth
- To ensure a full dose has been taken, repeat step 3 for a second time

**Step 4 Empty the inhaler**
- Open the outer lid and mouthpiece and discard the used capsule
- Wipe the mouthpiece clean and replace the cap

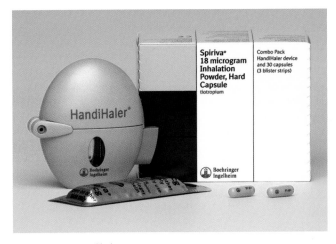

**Figure 9.11** A Handihaler.

## Breezhaler

The Breezhaler is a single-dose device which gives immediate feedback to indicate the dose has been taken correctly as the patient can hear a distinctive 'whirring' noise on inhalation (Figure 9.12). It delivers LAMA monotherapy, LABA monotherapy or LAMA and LABA in combination. It requires a capsule to be loaded into the device before use. These should never be swallowed and only capsules designed for use in a Breezhaler should be used (Box 9.13).

Box 9.13 **How to use a Breezhaler.**

**Step 1 Load the inhaler**
- Pull off the cap from the device
- To open the inhaler, hold the base firmly and tilt the mouthpiece open
- Separate one of the blisters from the blister card
- Peel away the protective backing to expose the capsule (do not push the capsule through the foil and only open the blister immediately before use)
- Remove the capsule and place into capsule chamber
- Close the mouthpiece firmly against the base until a click is heard

**Step 2 Pierce the capsule**
- Hold the Breezhaler with the mouthpiece pointed upwards
- Pierce the capsule by pressing both side buttons firmly at the same time (a click should be heard as the capsule is pierced)
- Release the side buttons fully
- Do not press the buttons more than once or shake the inhaler

**Step 3 Inhale the drug**
- Ensure the device is held horizontally with the side buttons to the left and right
- Hold the Breezhaler away from the mouth and exhale fully (take care not to breathe into the device)
- Place lips around the mouthpiece and ensure a good seal
- Breathe inwards quickly, deeply and fully (a whirring sound should be heard)
- Hold breath for up to 10 seconds or as long as is comfortable
- Remove the inhaler from the mouth
- Check a full dose has been taken by determining if powder remains in the capsule. If so, repeat step 3 for a second time

**Step 4 Empty the inhaler**
- Open the inhaler mouthpiece and discard the used capsule
- Wipe the mouthpiece clean and replace the cap

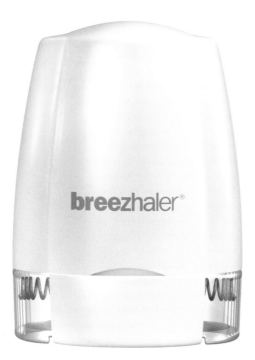

**Figure 9.12** A Breezhaler.

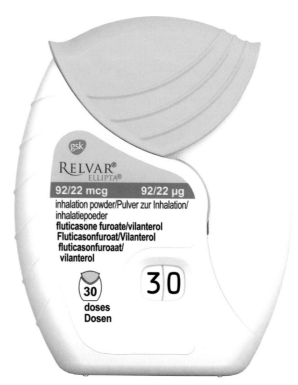

**Figure 9.13** An Ellipta.

## Ellipta

The Ellipta is a multidose device that delivers LAMA monotherapy, LAMA and LABA in combination or ICS and LABA in combination (Figure 9.13). It has a dose counter on the front that starts at 30, reduces to zero and displays red once 10 doses remain. After the last dose is used, half of the dose counter shows red and the number displays 0 (Box 9.14).

---

Box 9.14 **How to use an Ellipta.**

- Do not shake the inhaler
- Slide the cover down until a click is heard
- Ensure the dose counter reduces by 1 to confirm correct loading
- Hold the Ellipta away from the mouth and exhale fully (taking care not to breathe into the device)
- Place lips around the mouthpiece to ensure a tight seal (taking care not to block the air vent with fingers)
- Breathe inwards quickly, deeply and fully
- Hold breath for as long as possible (ideally at least 3–4 seconds)
- Remove the inhaler from the mouth
- Exhale gently
- Wipe the mouthpiece clean
- Close the inhaler by sliding the cover upwards

---

Box 9.15 **How to use a Genuair.**

- Remove the protective cap
- Hold the device with the mouthpiece towards you and the button at the back facing upwards (without tilting the inhaler)
- Depress the button completely and release it
- Ensure the colour control window has changed to green (this indicates the dose is ready for inhalation)
- Repeat the press and release action if the colour control window remains red
- Hold the device away from the mouth and exhale fully (taking care not to breathe into it)
- Place lips around the mouthpiece to ensure a good seal
- Breathe inwards quickly, deeply and fully
- Continue to inhale even after a click is heard (this indicates correct technique)
- Remove the inhaler from the mouth and hold breath for as long as comfortably possible
- Exhale slowly through the nose
- Ensure the colour control window has turned red (this confirms the dose has been taken). If it remains green, inhale strongly and deeply through the mouthpiece again
- Once the window has turned red, wipe the mouthpiece clean and replace the cap

---

## Genuair (Novoliser)

The Genuair is a multidose device that delivers LAMA monotherapy or LAMA and LABA in combination (Figure 9.14). To help establish when the device is empty, the Genuair has a dose counter above the colour control window; this starts at 60 and reduces to zero (Box 9.15). A red striped band appears in the dose window indicating that only a few doses remain. When the last dose has been prepared for inhalation, the button at the rear of the device will not return to its full upper position but will be locked in a middle position. Despite this, the last dose can be inhaled.

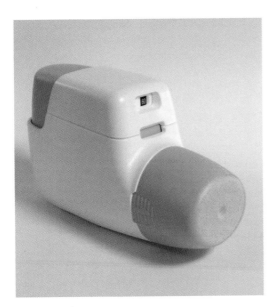

**Figure 9.14** A Genuair.

## Spiromax

The Spiromax is a multidose device which delivers ICS and LABA in combination (Figure 9.15). It has a dose counter at the rear of the device that starts at 60 and reduces to zero (Box 9.16). When

Box 9.16 **How to use a Spiromax.**

- Hold the inhaler upright with the mouthpiece facing you
- Open the mouthpiece cover by folding it down; a click should be heard indicating the inhaler is ready for use
- Hold the Spiromax away from the mouth and exhale fully (taking care not to breathe into the device)
- Place lips around the mouthpiece to ensure a good seal (taking care not to block the air vent with fingers)
- Breathe inwards quickly, deeply and fully
- Hold breath for 10 seconds or for as long as possible
- Remove the inhaler from the mouth and gently exhale
- Close the inhaler mouthpiece by folding it back up
- Repeat these steps if a second dose is required.
- Wipe the mouthpiece clean and replace the cap

20 doses remain, the numbers will appear in red but once zero is displayed in the window, the device is empty. The device will still click when the mouthpiece is opened even when empty.

## Nexthaler

The Nexthaler is a multidose device which delivers ICS and LABA in combination (Figure 9.16). It has a dose counter that starts at 120 and reduces to zero by one count each time (Box 9.17). A new

Box 9.17 **How to use a Nexthaler.**

- Hold the inhaler in an upright position
- Open the cover fully (a click should be heard)
- Hold the Nexthaler away from the mouth and breathe out fully (take care not to breathe into the device)

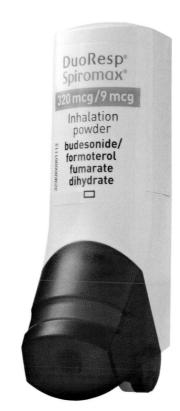

**Figure 9.15** A Spiromax.

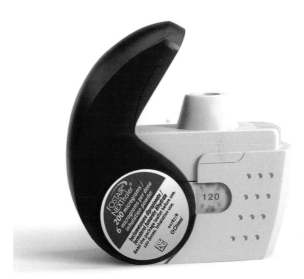

**Figure 9.16** A Nexthaler.

- Place lips around the mouthpiece to ensure a good seal (taking care not to block the air vent with fingers)
- Breathe inwards quickly, deeply and fully
- Hold breath for 10 seconds or for as long as possible
- Remove the inhaler from the mouth and gently exhale
- Move inhaler back to the upright position
- Close the cover fully
- Check the dose counter has gone down by 1
- Wipe the mouthpiece clean

inhaler is sealed within a protective pouch contained in a small box. After removal from the pouch, the new inhaler must be used within 6 months.

## Nebulisers

Nebulisers are usually driven by compressed air but can be driven by oxygen if the patient has no history of hypercapnic respiratory failure. They create a mist of drug particles, which is inhaled (during tidal breathing) via a facemask or mouthpiece. Despite lack of objective benefit compared to the use of a pMDI with spacer or DPI, many patients express confidence in nebulisers and believe them to be more effective than other methods of drug delivery, and they are often the preferred (and requested) option.

Determining which patients should be prescribed a nebuliser to deliver short acting bronchodilators in COPD is controversial. Indeed, with the introduction and increasing use of DPIs, the correct use of hand-held devices is possible for most patients. This in turn implies that fewer patients should be considered eligible for a domiciliary nebuliser. It is, however, reasonable to issue a nebuliser to patients with persistent and troublesome symptoms despite maximal treatment and good adherence to therapy and inhaler technique, although evidence of benefit should ideally be demonstrated. What actually qualifies as 'benefit' is far from clear, but may include a combination of reduction in breathlessness, improvement in exercise capacity, greater ability to perform daily living activities, reduced frequency of exacerbations and, perhaps especially, reduced hospital admissions. Another indication is complete inability to correctly use or co-ordinate hand-held devices. Individuals using a nebuliser should receive adequate training and a facility for appropriate servicing and support should be available. Portable hand-held nebulisers of varying performance – in terms of drug delivery – are now also available.

## Further reading

Broeders MEAC, Sanchis J, Levy ML, Crompton GK, Dekhuijzen PNR on behalf of the ADMIT Working Group. The ADMIT series – issues in inhalation therapy. 2) Improving technique and clinical effectiveness. *Primary Care Respiratory Journal* 2009; **18**: 76–82.

Chrystyn H, Small M, Milligan G, Higgins V, Garcia Gil E, Estruch J. Impact of patient satisfaction with their inhalers on treatment compliance and health status in COPD. *Respiratory Medicine* 2014; **108**: 358–365.

Jarvis S, Ind PW, Shiner RJ. Inhaled therapy in elderly COPD patients; time for re-evaluation? *Age and Ageing* 2007; **36**: 213–218.

Molimard M, Colthorpe P. Inhaler devices for chronic obstructive pulmonary disease: insights from patients and healthcare practitioners. *Journal of Aerosol Medicine and Pulmonary Drug Delivery* 2015; **28**: 219–228.

Newman SP. Inhaler treatment options in COPD. *European Respiratory Review* 2005; **14**: 102–108.

Restrepo RD, Alvarez MT, Wittnebel LD et al. Medication adherence issues in patients treated for COPD. *International Journal of Chronic Obstructive Pulmonary Disease* 2008; **3**: 371–384.

Sanchis J, Corrigan C, Levy ML, Viejo JL. Inhaler devices – from theory to practice. *Respiratory Medicine* 2013; **107**:495–502.

VinkenW, Dekhuijzen PNR, Barnes P on behalf of the ADMIT Working Group. The ADMIT series – issues in inhalation therapy. 4) How to choose inhaler devices for the treatment of COPD. *Primary Care Respiratory Journal* 2010; **19**: 10–20.

Yawn B, Colice G L, Hodder R. Practical aspects of inhaler use in the management of chronic obstructive pulmonary disease in the primary care setting. *International Journal of Chronic Obstructive Pulmonary Disease* 2012; **7**: 495–502.

# CHAPTER 10

# Surgical and Interventional Strategies

*James L. Lordan*

Freeman Hospital, University of Newcastle-upon-Tyne, UK

### OVERVIEW

- Interest in interventional approaches and transplantation has grown in recent years in patients with advanced chronic obstructive pulmonary disease (COPD) with persistent symptoms despite maximal treatment.
- Lung volume reduction (designed to remove poorly functioning areas of emphysematous lung) can be carried out surgically or less invasively by interventional bronchoscopists.
- Surgical lung volume reduction can be effective in patients with upper lobe emphysema and low exercise capacity.
- Bronchoscopic lung volume reduction can be performed using a variety of techniques; endobronchial valve and coil implantation have been studied most.
- Lung transplantation can be performed in carefully selected patients with functionally limiting advanced COPD; regional centre guidelines should be followed to determine when to refer.

Despite use of non-pharmacological and pharmacological manoeuvres, many patients continue to experience persistent and progressive symptoms of chronic obstructive pulmonary disease (COPD) with an associated decline in lung function. This in turn has led to greater interest in interventional and surgical approaches to management such as lung volume reduction surgery (LVRS), bronchoscopic lung volume reduction (BLVR) and transplantation, especially in those with advanced functionally limiting disease.

## Lung volume reduction strategies

Lung volume reduction surgery was proposed over 60 years ago as a method to remove non-functioning abnormal emphysematous lung parenchyma, to allow re-expansion of remaining structurally preserved lung. It was hypothesised that doing so would be associated with restoration of elastic lung recoil, reduced dynamic hyperinflation, airway closure and gas trapping, and that the reduction in total lung capacity and residual volume would improve overall respiratory mechanics and reduce symptoms. Lung volume reduction can be performed surgically or less invasively via a bronchoscope.

## Surgical lung volume reduction approaches

### Bullectomy

In some patients with COPD, bullae can occupy large volumes of the chest cavity, causing compression of surrounding functional lung parenchyma (Figure 10.1). Surgical excision of giant bullae can be associated with significant benefits (for example, in lung function and quality of life), particularly for large paraseptal bullae occupying more than one-third of the hemithorax. Bullectomy can also be considered in patients with previous pneumothorax or haemoptysis. Removal of giant bullae can now successfully be performed with video-assisted thoracoscopic surgery (VATS).

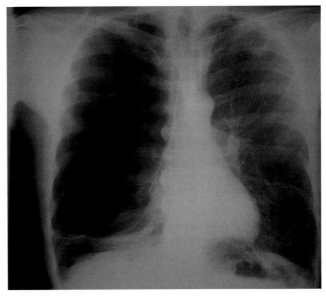

**Figure 10.1** A large right-sided lung bulla in a patient with chronic obstructive pulmonary disease.

---

*ABC of COPD*, Third Edition. Edited by Graeme P. Currie.
© 2017 John Wiley & Sons Ltd. Published 2017 by John Wiley & Sons Ltd.

## Lung volume reduction surgery

Lung volume reduction surgery involves removal of inefficient emphysematous lung parenchyma, allowing functioning lung tissue to re-expand, resulting in improved gas exchange. Initial LVRS attempts were associated with high perioperative mortality and little improvement in overall function. This in turn led on to the National Emphysema Treatment Trial (NETT) which studied outcomes in patients with COPD of different characteristics. This study explored the role of LRVS (performed by either median sternotomy or bilateral VATS) in COPD, with a median follow-up of 4.3 years, and randomised 1218 individuals ($FEV_1 <45\%$) with air trapping (residual volume >150%) and hyperinflation (total lung capacity >100%) to either LVRS or best medical care (including pulmonary rehabilitation).

The NETT failed to identify a survival advantage between medical or surgically treated patients. However, subgroup analysis demonstrated differing results depending on whether patients had upper versus non-upper predominant emphysema and low versus high baseline exercise capacity (Table 10.1). Those most likely to benefit (in terms of survival and improved exercise capacity) had upper lobe-predominant disease and low exercise capacity, while those with non-upper lobe-predominant emphysema with high exercise capacity experienced poorer survival versus conventional treatment. Findings from the NETT and other studies have helped identify which patients are more likely to benefit from LVRS.

**Table 10.1** Characteristic of patients likely to benefit and not benefit from surgical lung volume reduction surgery.

| Lower risk (better outcome) | High risk (poorer outcome/ contraindicated) |
|---|---|
| Age <75 years | DLCO <20% predicted |
| High MMRC dyspnoea score >3 | $FEV_1 <20\%$ |
| Severe emphysema ($FEV_1 <35\%$ predicted) | Pulmonary hypertension (PASP >35 mmHg) |
| TLC >125%, RV/TLC >0.65) | Coronary artery disease |
| Upper lobe-predominant emphysema | Homogeneous emphysema |
| Low exercise capacity | High exercise capacity |

DLCO, diffusing capacity of the lung for carbon monoxide; $FEV_1$, forced expiratory volume in 1 second; MMRC, modified Medical Research Council; PASP, pulmonary artery systolic pressure; RV, residual volume; TLC, total lung capacity.

## Bronchoscopic lung volume reduction strategies

Partly due to the relatively high perioperative risks and costs associated with LVRS, less invasive approaches using a bronchoscope have received increasing interest. Different strategies have been developed to achieve bronchoscopic lung volume reduction (BLVR); these include endobronchial valve (EBV) placement, lung volume reduction coil (LVRC) implantation, bronchoscopic thermal vapour ablation and polymeric lung volume reduction with air sealant (Table 10.2). These techniques differ in indication, mechanisms of action (airway 'blocking' versus 'non-blocking'), efficacy, complications and reversibility. No comparative trial between methods has been performed.

### Endobronchial valve placement

The most common BLVR technique is EBV implantation. One-way EBVs can be inserted into segmental airways of damaged lung parenchyma using a bronchoscope; these facilitate the exit of air and secretions on expiration, and block air entry on inhalation (Figures 10.2, 10.3). This dynamic process results in eventual segmental or lobar atelectasis and lung volume reduction. Complete lobar occlusion is an important endpoint to achieve clinical improvement with EBV. Two types of valves are available for clinical use: the EBV (Zephyr®, Pulmonx Corp, Redmond city, CA, USA) and intrabronchial valve (IBV) (Spiration®, Olympus, Tokyo, Japan). Both valves have similar mechanisms of action but different shapes.

One randomised controlled clinical trial in patients with heterogenous emphysema demonstrated statistically significant improvements in $FEV_1$, exercise tolerance and quality of life following placement of EBVs. In the same study, greatest benefit was found in those patients with complete interlobar fissures who achieved full lobar occlusion following EBV insertion. Patients with $FEV_1 <35\%$ and residual volume (RV) >200% predicted are considered likely to derive more benefit from EBV placement. It is usually avoided in patients requiring anticoagulation, due to the risk of haemoptysis. The presence of collateral ventilation (ventilation of alveolar structures through passages or channels that bypass the normal airways) is a contraindication to EBV placement, due to predicted clinical failure; its presence is determined by high-resolution computed tomography and use of the Chartis pulmonary assessment system.

**Table 10.2** Bronchoscopic lung volume reduction methods, indications and mechanisms of action.

| Method | Indication | Collateral ventilation dependence | Reversibility | Mechanism of action |
|---|---|---|---|---|
| Endobronchial valves | Upper or lower lobe emphysema | Yes | Yes (fully) | One-way occlusion of emphysema-damaged pulmonary lobe with atelectasis |
| Coils | Upper or lower lobe emphysema, homogeneous and heterogeneous emphysema | No | Partially reversible within first 4 weeks | Torquing of bronchi, compression of emphysema-damaged tissue, and volume loss |
| Bronchoscopic thermal vapour ablation | Upper lobe emphysema | No | Irreversible | Local instillation of water vapour (75 °C), inflammatory response, localised lobar fibrosis, and volume loss |
| Bypass tract airway stenting | Homogeneous emphysema | No | Irreversible | Stents placed endobronchially directly into emphysematous tissue |

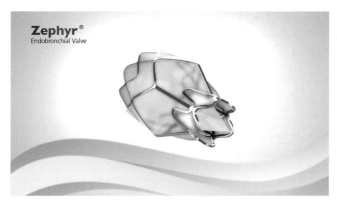

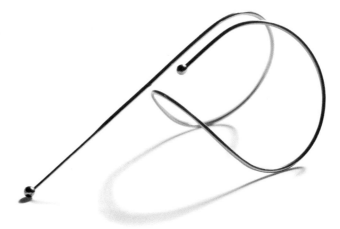

**Figure 10.2** An endobronchial valve.

**Figure 10.4** An endobronchial coil.

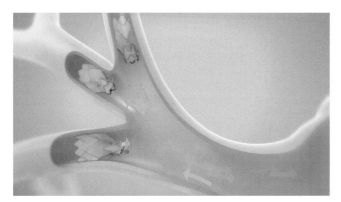

**Figure 10.3** Illustration of the functional properties of an endobronchial valve *in situ* on expiration and inspiration.

## Lung volume reduction coils

Bronchoscopic lung volume reduction can also be achieved using coils (RePneu®, PneumRx, Inc., Mountain View, CA, USA), which are independent of collateral ventilation (Figure 10.4). The shape-memory nitinol coils, designed to reduce hyperinflation and improve elastic recoil, can be delivered bronchoscopically under general anaesthetic. They can be placed in both lungs affected by upper or lower, heterogeneous or homogeneous emphysema and may lead to subsequent airway distortion and compression of diseased lung parenchyma. Some studies have shown significant clinical benefits in quality of life and exercise tolerance, although complications were noted early; complete removal of coils is not always possible, particularly after 4 weeks.

## Bronchoscopic thermal vapour ablation

Bronchoscopic thermal vapour ablation is a method whereby localised thermal injury is induced following airway injection of water vapour to areas of damaged lung parenchyma. This causes fibrosis, scar formation and regional lung volume reduction. The technique is irreversible, independent of collateral ventilation, and can be considered in some patients with persistent symptoms, advanced airflow obstruction and predominantly upper lobe emphysema. Some studies have shown improvements in quality of life and lung function with an acceptable safety profile.

## Biological lung volume reduction

Biological lung volume reduction can be achieved by the instillation of a fibrinogen-based biopharmaceutical suspension. This polymerises in the target airways to form a biodegradable matrix, with subsequent localised inflammatory response inducing distal fibrosis, collapse and volume reduction of the target lobar segment. The role of this technique requires further evaluation.

## Endobronchial and extrapulmonary bypass procedures

Airway bypass procedures have been proposed as a strategy to treat homogeneous emphysema. This creates extra-anatomical fenestrated airway channels using a needle-tipped catheter to form connections between segmental airways and emphysematous lung parenchymal tissue to achieve greater exhalation and LVR. Further studies are required.

## Lung transplantation

Lung transplantation is a widely accepted therapeutic option for selected patients with end-stage respiratory disease, such as COPD and α1-antitrypsin deficiency (α1-ATD) related emphysema, who fail to satisfactorily respond to conventional approaches. It is primarily performed for survival benefit, although significant improvements in quality of life are achieved for the majority of recipients. Careful candidate selection and optimisation of treatment are vital to guide timing of referral and listing for transplantation, and to identify patients most likely to benefit.

Approximately 40% of lung transplants are performed worldwide for COPD (33%) and α1-ATD-related emphysema (6%) (Figures 10.5, 10.6).

### Patient selection

Individuals with α1-ATD present earlier with severe disease, but have less co-morbidity and therefore a better post-transplant outcome than those with COPD. Due to the variable course of COPD, difficulty exists in precisely identifying criteria associated with a survival benefit from transplantation. Evaluation of a patient's biological age and physical and mental 'robustness' is important; older

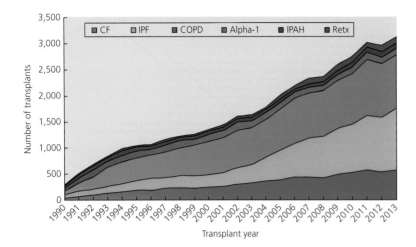

**Figure 10.5** Number of transplants according to transplant year for different indications. Abbreviations: CF: cystic fibrosis, IPF: idiopathic pulmonary fibrosis, COPD: chronic obstructive pulmonary disease, Alpha-1: Alpha-1 antitrypsin deficiency, IPAH: idiopathic pulmonary arterial hypertension, Retx: retransplantation. Reproduced with permission from ISHLT Registry data 2015.

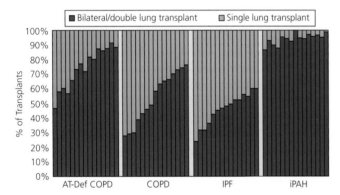

**Figure 10.6** Increasing trend for bilateral lung transplantation, compared to single lung transplantion for different indications including α1-antitrypsin deficiency (a-ATDef COPD), chronic obstructive pulmonary disease (COPD), idiopathic pulmonary fibrosis (IPF) and idiopathic pulmonary arterial hypertension (iPAH). Reproduced with permission from ISHLT Registry data 2015.

- Chest wall deformity/pump disorders (e.g. severe kyphoscoliosis, neuromuscular disorders or diaphragm dysfunction)
- Body mass index >35 (ideally >18 and <30)
- Poor adherence to medical care
- Psychiatric or psychological disease likely to affect long-term outcome
- Inadequate social support
- Physical frailty with poor rehabilitation potential
- Active substance abuse or dependency (alcohol, cigarettes, nicotine or illicit substances)

patients (>65 years) have a less favourable outcome following lung transplantation due to increased co-morbid disease adversely influencing post-transplant recovery. The International Society of Heart and Lung Transplantation has published criteria which outline absolute and relative contraindications to transplantation, including COPD-specific referral and listing criteria (Boxes 10.1, 10.2).

> **Box 10.1 Absolute contraindications to lung transplantation.**
>
> - Previous malignancy (5-year disease-free interval recommended for haematological malignancies, sarcoma, melanoma or solid organ cancers, while a 2-year interval considered, for skin malignancy at low recurrence risk)
> - Irreversible organ dysfunction (e.g. brain, cardiac, renal or liver).
> - Coronary artery disease, not suitable for revascularisation, atherosclerosis-related end-organ disease
> - Active or recurrent sepsis
> - Uncorrectable bleeding diathesis
> - Active or inadequately controlled chronic infection (e.g. *Mycobacterium tuberculosis*)

> **Box 10.2 Relative contraindications to lung transplantation; the presence of one absolute or a number of relative contraindications may preclude lung transplantation.**
>
> - Age >65 with co-morbidities
> - Body mass index 30–35
> - Progressive cachexia (body mass index <18) unresponsive to supplementation, gastrostomy or nasogastric feeding
> - Severe, symptomatic osteoporosis (particularly if fractures)
> - Previous thoracic surgery with pleuropulmonary adhesions or mediastinal shift
> - Mechanical ventilation
> - Highly virulent bacteria/fungal infections (e.g. mycetomas or mycobacteria, in particular *M. abscessus*)
> - Hepatitis B or C (considered in the absence of cirrhosis, portal hypertension, absent virus replication by selected centres)
> - Human immunodeficiency virus (considered if controlled, virus undetectable and compliant with antiretroviral therapy)

Previous thoracic surgery is not uncommon in patients referred for lung transplantation; LVRS or previous pneumothorax managed by intercostal drainage or pleurodesis is not a contraindication. LVR (surgically or bronchoscopically) can be performed prior to consideration of transplantation.

## Timing of listing for transplantation

Various criteria have been suggested to aid timing of referral and listing for transplantation (Boxes 10.3, 10.4). An intrinsic shortage of donor organs can lead to a prolonged wait time for transplantation, despite attempts to increase organ donation and the pool of available donor lungs. Bridging strategies can be implemented for patients declining rapidly on the transplant waiting list, such as domiciliary nocturnal bi-level positive airway pressure (BiPAP) with oxygen supplementation. Highly selected patients can be considered for advanced intensive care-based support measures as a bridge to transplantation, although this is less commonly implemented in patients with COPD due to co-morbid factors and older recipient age. However, younger fitter patients with severe hypercapnic respiratory failure can be supported with a Novalung® (lung assist device, LAD) to help with oxygen delivery and $CO_2$ elimination in an attempt to avoid intubation. Extracorporeal membrane oxygenation (ECMO) has also been used to bridge patients to transplantation.

---

**Box 10.3 International Society of Heart and Lung Transplantation consensus recommendations for assessment and listing patients with COPD and α1-ATD for lung transplantation.**

**When to refer for assessment**

- Evidence of disease progression, despite maximum medical and interventional treatment
- Candidate not suitable for surgical or endoscopic lung volume reduction intervention
- BODE index 5–6
- $PaCO_2 > 6.6\,kPa$ and/or $PaO_2 < 8\,kPa$
- $FEV_1 < 25\%$ predicted

**When to consider listing for transplant**

- BODE index ≥7
- $FEV_1 < 15–20\%$ predicted
- Frequent severe exacerbations requiring hospital admission
- Severe exacerbations with hypercapnic respiratory failure requiring non-invasive ventilation
- Moderate-to-severe pulmonary artery hypertension

---

**Box 10.4 Factors associated with increased mortality in COPD and α1-antitrypsin deficiency.**

- Older age
- Lower body mass index
- High dyspnoea score
- Supplemental oxygen requirement
- Reduced 6-minute walk distance
- Low $VO_2$ max

---

- Lower $FEV_1$ (<30%)
- Higher residual volume
- Lower DLCO
- Hypoxaemia
- Hyercapnia or hypocapnia
- Lower haemoglobin
- Lower lobe-predominant emphysema
- Pulmonary hypertension
- Frequent exacerbations requiring hospital admission
- Single exacerbation with hypercapnia
- High BODE index

BODE, body mass index, airflow obstruction, dyspnoea and exercise capacity; DLCO, diffusing capacity of the lung for carbon monoxide; $FEV_1$, forced expiratory volume in 1 second; $VO_2$ max, a measure of oxygen consumption.

---

## Post-transplant management, complications and survival

Bilateral lung transplant is the preferred procedure for COPD, although single lung transplant can be considered for older patients with co-morbidities when a bilateral procedure may not be tolerated. Following transplantation, important considerations include:

- triple immunosuppression regimens, such as with a calcineurin inhibitor (ciclosporin or tacrolimus), a cell cycle inhibitor (azathioprine or mycophenolate mofetil), and tapering oral corticosteroids
- post-transplant surveillance, such as perioperative antimicrobial prophylaxis, lifelong *Pneumocystis jirovecii* pneumonia prophylaxis (co-trimoxazole), herpes (aciclovir) and selected cytomegalovirus surveillance (valganciclovir)
- regular fibreoptic bronchoscopy with transbronchial biopsy and microbiology cultures (to ensure good lung allograft function, allow inspection of bronchial anastomosis and identify and treat acute vascular rejection or infection)
- encouraging adherence to drugs
- availability of a robust social support network
- provision of a patient education programme.

Regular transplant team and local clinician follow-up are vital following lung transplantation. As well as providing an opportunity for education, they help identify the development of complications (Table 10.3, Figure 10.7).

## Summary

Exciting developments have taken place in recent years exploring less invasive interventional and surgical treatments for the management of advanced symptomatic COPD. Transplantation for COPD continues to increase worldwide, although limited by donor lung availability, with improved functional and survival outcomes, particularly in large-volume centres. Further research and development in organ preservation technology, stem cell, matrix scaffolding and recellularising tissue bioengineering, an increased understanding of

**Table 10.3** Early and late complications following lung transplantation.

| | Complication | Treatment |
|---|---|---|
| Early | Primary graft dysfunction | Supportive treatment |
| | Acute rejection | Corticosteroid augmentation and taper |
| | Surgery-related infection | Surgical drainage and antimicrobial therapy |
| | Pulmonary vascular complications | Early identification and surgical revision |
| | Bronchial anastomosis dehiscence | Early surgical revision |
| | Drug toxicity/adverse effects (e.g. nephrotoxicity, myelosuppression, neurotoxicity) | Adjustment in immunosuppression regimen or dose adjustment |
| | Adverse drug interactions | |
| | Infection due to immunosuppression | Optimal antimicrobial therapy |
| Late | Post-transplant lymphoproliferative disorders | Immunosuppression intensity reduction, may require rituximab or chemotherapy |
| | Malignancy (skin cancer, lung cancer) | Regular dermatology surveillance, sun avoidance and smoking cessation |
| | Chronic lung allograft dysfunction (bronchiolitis obliterans syndrome and restrictive allograft syndrome) | Azithromycin/photophoresis/total lymphoid irradiation/oesophageal fundoplication |
| | Drug toxicity/adverse effects (nephrotoxicity, myelosuppression, neurotoxicity) | Therapeutic trough level, blood monitoring, and tailoring of immunosuppression regimen |
| | Adverse drug interactions | Awareness of potential interactions |
| | Infection due to immunosuppression | Inhaled or oral antimicrobial prophylaxis |
| | Renal dysfunction | Calcineurin level optimisation |
| | Diabetes mellitus | Diet, insulin or oral hypoglycaemic agent |
| | Hyperlipidaemia | Atorvastatin, as statin of choice |
| | Hypertension | |

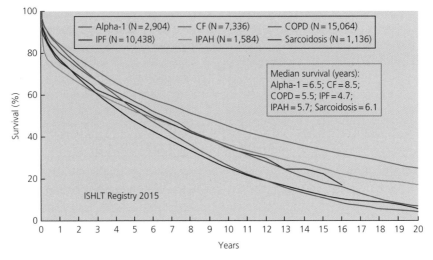

**Figure 10.7** Life expectancy post transplant for different indications. Abbreviations: Alpha-1: Alpha-1 antitrypsin deficiency, CF: cystic fibrosis, COPD: chronic obstructive pulmonary disease, IPF: idiopathic pulmonary fibrosis, IPAH: idiopathic pulmonary arterial hypertension. Reproduced with permission from ISHLT Registry data 2015.

alloimmune tolerance and less toxic immuno-suppressive regimens are required. This will hopefully revolutionise the outcome for patients with COPD requiring organ support or transplantation.

## Further reading

Eberhardt R, Gompelmann D, Herth FJ, Schuhmann M. Endoscopic bronchial valve treatment: patient selection and special considerations. *International Journal of Chronic Obstructive Pulmonary Disorder* 2015; **10**: 2147–2157.

Hartert M, Senbaklavacin O, Gohrbandt B, Fischer BM, Buhl R, Vahld CF. Lung transplantation: a treatment option in end-stage lung disease. *Deutsches Arzteblatt International* 2014; **111**: 107–16.

Lane CR, Tonelli AR. Lung transplantation in chronic obstructive pulmonary disease: patient selection and special considerations. *International Journal of Chronic Obstructive Pulmonary Disorder* 2015; **10**: 2137–2146.

Trotter MA, Hopkins PM. Advanced therapies for COPD – what's on the horizon? Progress in lung volume reduction and lung transplantation. *Journal of Thoracic Disease* 2014; **6**: 1640–1653.

Vos R, Verleden SE, Verleden GM. Chronic lung allograft dysfunction: evolving practice. *Current Opinion in Organ Transplantation* 2015; **20**: 483–491.

Weill D, Benden C, Corris PA et al. A consensus document for the selection of lung transplant candidates: 2014 – an update from the Pulmonary Transplantation Council of the International Society for Heart and Lung Transplantation. *Journal of Heart and Lung Transplantation* 2015; **34**: 1–15.

Yusen RD, Edwards LB, Kucheryavaya AY et al. The Registry of the International Society for Heart and Lung Transplantation: Thirty-second Official Adult Lung and Heart-Lung Transplantation Report--2015; Focus Theme: Early Graft Failure. *Journal of Heart and Lung Transplantation* 2015; **34**: 1264–1277.

# CHAPTER 11

# Oxygen

*Graham Douglas, Margaret Macleod and Graeme P. Currie*

Aberdeen Royal Infirmary, Aberdeen, UK

## OVERVIEW

- Normal oxygen saturation is between 95% and 98% in healthy adults breathing air at sea level.

- Pulse oximeters are portable, non-invasive devices which assess oxygen saturation ($SpO_2$).

- An oxygen saturation ≤92% can be used to identify patients who may require home oxygen assessment, or ≤94% where there is peripheral oedema, polycythaemia or pulmonary hypertension.

- Giving high concentrations of oxygen to hypercapnic patients with COPD can lead to hypoventilation, a rise in $PaCO_2$ and development of acidosis.

- The target $SpO_2$ is 88–92% during an exacerbation of chronic obstructive pulmonary disease (COPD); reduce the inspired oxygen concentration if $SpO_2$ rises to >92%.

- In hospital, for patients with COPD who have normal pH and $PaCO_2$, the target $SpO_2$ is 94–98%.

- Long-term oxygen therapy (LTOT) is beneficial in patients with resting $PaO_2$ on air ≤7.3 kPa on two separate occasions when stable, or those with $PaO_2$ 7.3–8 kPa with secondary polycythaemia (haematocrit ≥55%), pulmonary hypertension, peripheral oedema or nocturnal hypoxaemia.

- Ambulatory oxygen may be helpful to patients who are shown to desaturate on exertion; it can be delivered by a small lightweight oxygen cylinder, liquid oxygen system or portable oxygen concentrator.

- Conserving devices or demand flow valves allow delivery of oxygen during inspiration only; this facilitates use of smaller, more portable cylinders with increased usage time and reduced cost of oxygen delivery.

- There is little evidence that breathless patients with COPD benefit from short-burst oxygen.

- In COPD patients considering air travel, oxygen is not required if $SpO_2$ on air is >95% but is advised if $SpO_2$ is <92%; those with $SpO_2$ 92–95% should ideally have a hypoxic challenge test (breathing 15% oxygen).

In patients with chronic obstructive pulmonary disease (COPD), oxygen is used in a variety of settings. For example, it can be used at home (at rest and/or only on exertion), during transport to and from hospital and in hospital during an exacerbation. Administering oxygen is not without its dangers and it should usually be prescribed like any other drug, taking into account potential hazards or risks such as smoking, vicinity of naked flames and risk of tripping over lengthy oxygen tubing.

Prescription should indicate when and for how long it should be used. Specify separate ambulatory and long-term oxygen therapy (LTOT) flow rates for each patient, as different rates may be required. All medical staff, nursing staff and ambulance crews should be aware of the dangers of injudicious use of oxygen. At all times, therefore, consider whether oxygen is actually necessary.

## Oxygen physiology

Most circulating oxygen is bound to haemoglobin. As there is a fixed amount of haemoglobin, the amount of oxygen carried is usually expressed as the 'oxygen saturation' of haemoglobin. From an arterial sample, this is called $SaO_2$ and from a pulse oximeter, $SpO_2$. Alternatively, the oxygen tension or 'partial pressure of oxygen' ($PaO_2$) can be measured from an arterial sample of blood. The oxygen dissociation curve shows the relationship between oxygen saturation and arterial oxygen pressure (Figure 11.1). In healthy adults at sea level with normal $PaO_2$, $SpO_2$ is maintained between 95% and 98%.

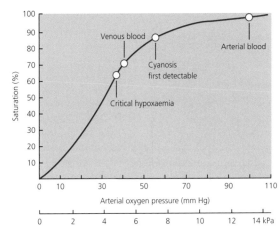

**Figure 11.1** The oxygen dissociation curve.

*ABC of COPD*, Third Edition. Edited by Graeme P. Currie.
© 2017 John Wiley & Sons Ltd. Published 2017 by John Wiley & Sons Ltd.

## Pulse oximetry

An oximeter is a spectrophotometric device that measures $SpO_2$ by determining the differential absorption of light by oxyhaemoglobin and deoxyhaemoglobin (Figure 11.2). Modern oximeters use a probe incorporating a light source and sensor that can be attached to the patient's finger or ear lobe. They are easy to use, portable, non-invasive and relatively inexpensive. There is a short delay of 30 seconds in registration due to circulation time and they are less accurate at $SpO_2$ levels below 75%.

Pulse oximeters should be available to assess all breathless or acutely ill patients in both primary and secondary care, although caution is required in interpretation in some circumstances (Table 11.1).

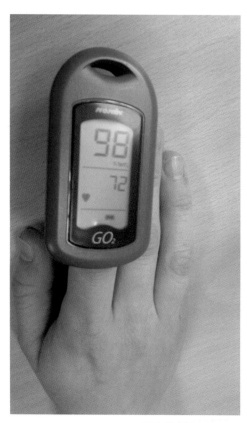

**Figure 11.2** A pulse oximeter.

**Table 11.1** Situations where measurement of $SpO_2$ with a pulse oximeter can lead to erroneous readings.

| Clinical situation | Result |
| --- | --- |
| Jaundice/hyperbilirubinaemia | Falsely low saturation |
| Movement (e.g. shivering) | Poor signal |
| Methaemoglobinaemia | Low level |
| Thickened skin due to callous | Poor signal |
| CO poisoning/high carboxyhaemoglobin | Falsely high saturation |
| Poor peripheral perfusion/hypothermia | Poor signal |
| Nail varnish | Poor signal |

## Oxygen during exacerbations of COPD

Some patients with advanced COPD (or during an exacerbation) have a fall in $PaO_2$ to <8 kPa and rise in $PaCO_2$; this is termed hypercapnic or type 2 respiratory failure. The underlying mechanism is complex but includes ventilation/perfusion mismatch, reduced buffering capacity of haemoglobin, absorption atelectasis and reduced ventilatory drive. Administrating high concentrations of oxygen in this situation can lead to diminished ventilation with further rise in $PaCO_2$ and development of a respiratory acidosis (pH <7.35), particularly if $PaO_2$ rises above 10 kPa. Indeed, many patients with COPD are 'acclimatised' to living with $SpO_2$ much lower than normal and are unlikely to benefit from a large increase in inspired oxygen even during an acute illness. In a large UK study of patients admitted to hospital with an exacerbation of COPD, as many as 47% had $PaCO_2$ >6.0 kPa, 20% had respiratory acidosis (pH <7.35) and 5% had severe acidosis (pH <7.25).

Patients with severe COPD and previous episodes of acute hypercapnic respiratory failure should therefore be given a personalised oxygen alert card (Figure 11.3) and Venturi valve and mask (24% or 28%) (Figures 11.4, 11.5) to help avoid inadvertent and potentially fatal administration of high concentrations of oxygen.

## Prehospital oxygen

Prior to initiation of oxygen, patients should show their oxygen alert card to the ambulance crew. A 28% Venturi mask at 4 L/min or 24% Venturi mask at 2 L/min, aiming for $SpO_2$ of 88–92%, should ideally be used in the community and during transport to hospital. The oxygen concentration should be reduced if $SpO_2$ exceeds 92% since this could lead to progressive $CO_2$ retention. If nebulised bronchodilators are administered, they should be given by compressed air and supplemental oxygen provided through nasal cannulae at a flow rate of 1–4 L/min.

## Hospital oxygen

As soon as possible after arrival in hospital, perform an arterial blood gas measurement. If pH and $PaCO_2$ are normal, aim for $SpO_2$ of 94–98% but if not, continue to aim for target $SpO_2$ of 88–92%. Recheck arterial blood gases 30–60 minutes after starting oxygen (or altering its concentration) to confirm that $PaCO_2$ has not increased.

Once patients are stable, consider changing from a Venturi mask to nasal cannulae at 1–2 L/min. Nasal cannulae (Figure 11.6) provide a variable fraction of inspired oxygen ($FiO_2$) depending on the flow rate and patient's minute volume, inspiratory flow and pattern of breathing. Rechecking arterial blood gases when the patient is stable on nasal cannulae is advisable.

## Long-term oxygen therapy

Two randomised controlled trials have shown that using oxygen for at least 15 hours each day improves survival and quality of life in hypoxaemic patients with COPD. Use of continuous oxygen

**OXYGEN ALERT CARD**

Name

I am at risk of type II respiratory failure with a raised $CO_2$ level. Please use my _____ % Venturi mask to achieve an oxygen saturation of _____ % to _____ % during exacerbations.

Use compressed air to drive nebulisers (with nasal oxygen at 2 l/min). If compressed air not available, limit oxygen-driven nebulisers to 6 minutes.

British Thoracic Society  COLLEGE OF **paramedics**
leading the development of the paramedic profession

— **OXYGEN ALERT CARD** —

The Intensive Care Society

**Figure 11.3** An example of an oxygen alert card. Source: courtesy of the British Thoracic Society.

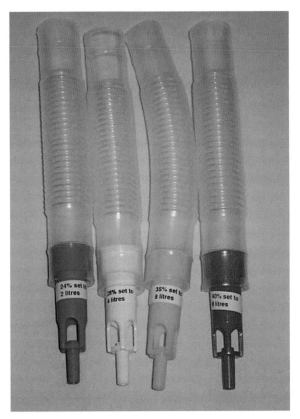

24% set to 2 litres   28% set to 4 litres   35% set to 8 litres   40% set to 8 litres

**Figure 11.4** A range of Venturi valves are available to deliver specific concentrations of oxygen at a given flow rate (24%, 28%, 35% and 40% are shown).

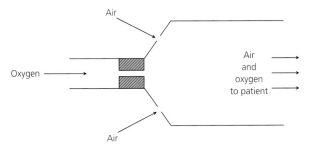

Air

Oxygen

Air and oxygen to patient

Air

**Figure 11.5** A Venturi valve plus mask mixes 100% oxygen at a given flow rate with room air (determined by the size of the ports in the valve). This produces a predictable concentration of oxygen in the facemask which is then delivered to the patient.

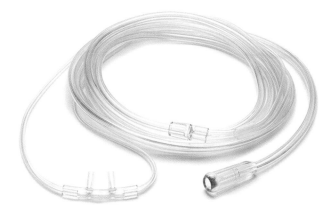

**Figure 11.6** Delivering oxygen through nasal cannulae enables patients to eat, drink and communicate more easily than with a full facemask. Source: courtesy of Vivisol Home Care Services.

therapy (24 hours) offers additional survival benefit compared to shorter durations. Consider LTOT in non-smoking patients with COPD if:

- $PaO_2 \leq 7.3$ kPa on two separate occasions at least 3 weeks apart during a period of clinical stability (ideally at least 8 weeks following an exacerbation), or
- $PaO_2$ is $\leq 8$ kPa and there is evidence of secondary polycythaemia (haematocrit $\geq 55\%$), pulmonary hypertension, peripheral oedema or nocturnal hypoxaemia.

Survival benefits have not been observed in patients with $PaO_2$ of 7.3–8.0 kPa without secondary complications or those who do not use LTOT for a minimum of 15 hours each day. Before arranging LTOT, ensure patients have stopped smoking and are aware of the dangers of naked flames in the proximity of oxygen delivery devices. Discuss smoking cessation (including stopping e-cigarette use) and provide written education to all patients prior to ordering home oxygen. Patients who continue to smoke while receiving home oxygen have poorer outcomes.

Long-term oxygen therapy is most conveniently and economically given by a concentrator that removes nitrogen from the air and supplies oxygen-enriched air (Figure 11.7). Nasal cannulae are the most practical means of delivering LTOT, although some patients may prefer a facemask, especially those with troublesome dry nasal mucosa. Although Venturi masks are commonly used in

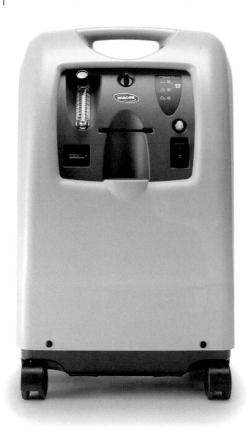

**Figure 11.7** A concentrator is the most convenient way to supply long-term oxygen to patients at home. A contractor supplies all oxygen in the UK. A prescription is sent from the specialist home oxygen assessment team requesting installation of appropriate equipment. Source: courtesy of Vivisol Home Care Services.

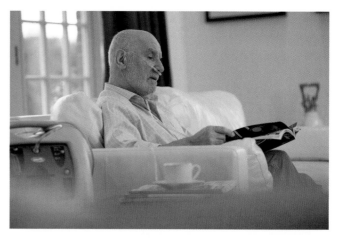

**Figure 11.8** Most patients prescribed LTOT can perform daily living activities within their home providing they have sufficiently long oxygen tubing and use nasal cannulae. Source: courtesy of Vivisol Home Care Services.

hospital and emergency care settings, they are usually incompatible with home concentrators as backpressure created in the tubing can damage the machine. Provide patients started on LTOT with formal education by a specialist home oxygen assessment team and review patients on at least an annual basis to ensure their oxygen prescription remains appropriate.

Patients should not normally have LTOT ordered at the time of an acute exacerbation. If it is supplied on discharge (e.g. for individuals who remain breathless with $SpO_2 \leq 88\%$ and when oxygen is difficult to wean), advise them that home oxygen might be removed if reassessment, once clinically stable, demonstrates improvement. Formal LTOT assessment should typically occur at least 8 weeks from their last exacerbation.

## Ambulatory oxygen

Ambulatory oxygen therapy (AOT) is the use of supplemental oxygen during exercise or activity. The necessity for AOT is based on measurement of $SpO_2$ using a pulse oximeter to identify desaturation on exercise plus any response to supplemental oxygen. Consider factors such as ability to carry cylinders and whether or not patients are mobile as part of the overall assessment. Providing AOT to suitable patients should aim to promote activities of daily living, greater independence and improved quality of life. Its usefulness, however, can be limited by the duration of oxygen

supply from a portable-sized cylinder that some patients may also find difficult to carry. Patients will require assessment for specific devices such as pulsed and liquid oxygen to ensure their inspiratory flow rate can trigger the demand flow valve. They should also be sufficiently "robust" to enable them to carry oxygen and have manual dexterity to manipulate the equipment.

Continuous flow of oxygen from a portable oxygen cylinder is reliable but very wasteful. About two-thirds of the supplied oxygen is wasted as the patient exhales. Oxygen-conserving devices, such as reservoir cannulae and demand pulsing devices, provide flow during inspiration but not during expiration. This leads to increased usage time, smaller cylinders and reduced cost of oxygen delivery.

A modern portable cylinder without an oxygen-conserving device will only last for up to 4 hours with a flow rate of 2 L/min and up to 2 hours with a flow rate of 4 L/min. Pulsed oxygen can last 2–3 times longer depending on the device and respiratory rate. AOT may be facilitated from a concentrator within the home using long tubing allowing the patient to move around their home, although care should be taken to avoid the associated trip hazard (Figure 11.8). In some areas of the UK, contractors will supply home filling cylinders that have a built-in conserving device or demand valve and can be filled at home by the patient (Figure 11.9). Backpacks are often used to carry ambulatory oxygen cylinders. In some circumstances (i.e. when dealing with less physically capable patients), however, it is easier and more practical to provide trolleys or carts. During transport in cars, cylinders should be secured with a seatbelt or placed in the footwell or car boot.

Liquid oxygen is increasingly used as a portable option for patients with COPD (Figure 11.10). Oxygen exists in a liquid state at temperatures below −180 °C and 30 litres of liquid will provide 25 000 litres of gas. There are specific risks associated with liquid oxygen, including cold burns, leakage and problems with installation of a reservoir unit above ground-floor level; liquid oxygen should therefore only be prescribed after a home risk assessment. It should always be transported in an upright position. A small portable flask can be filled quickly from the reservoir unit, providing an instant source of ambulatory oxygen as and when required. Portable oxygen concentrators are also becoming available for specific situations that may, for example, permit patients to go on holiday more easily or continue in employment.

## Short-burst oxygen

Despite maximal inhaled and oral pharmacological treatment, some patients with advanced COPD experience severe breathlessness on exertion. Studies in patients who do not fulfil the arterial blood gas criteria for prescription of LTOT generally demonstrate that oxygen after exercise fails to influence breathlessness scores or rate of symptomatic recovery. Oxygen used in this way may reduce the degree of dynamic hyperinflation during recovery from exercise, but fails to significantly alter the degree of breathlessness. Short-burst oxygen therapy has been described as 'one of the most expensive therapies used in the NHS' (BTS/NICE COPD Guidelines 2010) and should not generally be used prior to, or following, exercise. Where breathlessness continues in the absence of hypoxia, explore other causes and tailor strategies as indicated.

## Air travel and oxygen

Increasing numbers of individuals at extremes of age and with a variety of medical problems such as COPD and other chronic respiratory disorders are travelling by air. Commercial aircraft fly at 27 000–37 000 feet (9000–11 000 m) and are required to maintain cabin pressure at the equivalent of 8000 feet (2438 m). At this pressure, inspired oxygen is the equivalent of breathing 15% oxygen and therefore even in healthy subjects, $SpO_2$ falls. In patients with COPD, oxygenation may fall, causing breathlessness, which will be exacerbated by minimal exercise. Neither forced expiratory volume in 1 second ($FEV_1$) nor oxygen saturation ($SpO_2$), however, is able to predict development of hypoxia or complications arising during air travel.

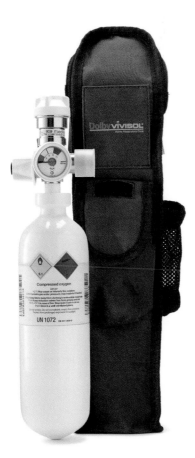

**Figure 11.9** An example of a homefill cylinder and compressor. Source: courtesy of Vivisol Home Care Services.

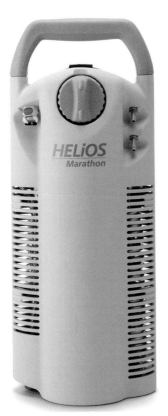

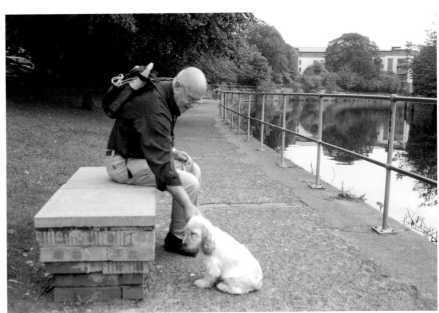

**Figure 11.10** Liquid oxygen is provided in a smaller container compared to conventional oxygen cylinders; a range of differently sized flasks are available. Source: courtesy of Vivisol Home Care Services.

## Who needs to be assessed?

Most patients with COPD fly in commercial aircraft without incident. Individuals with COPD who are otherwise well with $SpO_2 > 95\%$ on air generally do not require in-flight oxygen. British Thoracic Society guidelines advise medical assessment if there is doubt about fitness to fly or if the following characteristics are present:

- significant respiratory symptoms with previous air travel
- $FEV_1 < 30\%$ predicted
- severe restrictive lung disease (forced vital capacity <1 litre), especially if hypercapnia and hypoxia are present
- bullous lung disease
- existing requirement for home oxygen
- recent pneumothorax
- less than 6 weeks since hospital discharge for an acute respiratory illness.

Assessment should usually include history, examination and measurement of resting $SpO_2$. In some patients, a hypoxic challenge test may be required (if available locally) (Table 11.2).

## Hypoxic challenge testing

A hypoxic challenge test involves patients breathing 15% oxygen at sea level for 20 minutes to mimic the environment to which they would be exposed during a typical commercial flight – this may be facilitated using 100% nitrogen delivered via a 40% Venturi mask. Those with $PaO_2 \geq 6.6\,kPa$ ($SpO_2 \geq 85\%$) are considered not to require in-flight oxygen, while those with $PaO_2$ falling to <6.6 kPa ($SpO_2 < 85\%$) should have it arranged during the flight. In-flight oxygen can be prescribed at a rate of 2 or 4 L/min and is given by nasal cannulae. In some airlines, oxygen is delivered by a breath-activated system that may cause problems in those with poor respiratory reserve.

All patients with COPD who require in-flight oxygen should inform the relevant airline when booking and be aware that some airlines charge for this service. The need for oxygen while changing flights must also be considered and many airports can provide

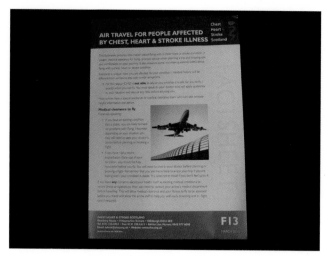

**Figure 11.11** Factsheets along with other sources of information (such ashttps://www.caa.co.uk/Passengers/Before-you-fly/Am-I-fit-to-fly-/) can be accessed which provide support and practical help for individuals with respiratory-related (and other) disabilities planning to travel by aircraft.

wheelchairs for transport to and from aircraft and within terminal buildings. Advise patients to carry both preventive and reliever inhalers in hand luggage; nebulisers may be used at the discretion of the in-flight crew and airline. Although inhaled bronchodilators are usually available in emergency airline medical kits, nebulisers are not. Other practical factors should also be considered such as having adequate medical insurance, requesting an aisle seat near to toilets, minimising alcohol intake, ensuring adequate oral hydration and need for a supply of rescue antibiotics and oral corticosteroids to take on holiday (Figure 11.11).

## Further reading

British Thoracic Society. BTS guidelines for home oxygen use in adults. *Thorax* 2015; **70**: i1–43.

Medical Research Council Working Party, Flenley DC. Long-term domiciliary oxygen therapy in chronic hypoxic cor pulmonale complicating chronic bronchitis and emphysema. *Lancet* 1981; **1**(8222): 681–686.

Nocturnal Oxygen Therapy Trial Group. Continuous or nocturnal oxygen therapy in hypoxemic chronic obstructive lung disease: a clinical trial. *Annals of Internal Medicine* 1980; **93**: 391–398.

Plant PK, Owen JL, Elliot MW. One year period prevalence study of respiratory acidosis in acute exacerbations of COPD: implications for the provision of non-invasive ventilation and oxygen administration. *Thorax* 2000; **55**: 550–554.

Stevenson NS, Calverley PMA. Effect of oxygen on recovery from maximal exercise in patients with COPD. *Thorax* 2004; **59**: 668–672.

www.brit-thoracic.org.uk/document-library/clinical-information/air-travel/bts-air-travel-recommendations-2011/

www.caa.co.uk/Passengers/Before-you-fly/Am-I-fit-to-fly/Guidance-for-health-professionals/Assessing-fitness-to-fly/

**Table 11.2** Advice regarding necessity of in-flight oxygen in commercial aircraft.

| Oxygen saturation on air | Recommendation |
|---|---|
| >95% | Oxygen not required |
| 92–95% (without risk factor*) | Oxygen not required |
| 92–95% (with risk factor*) | Hypoxic challenge test |
| <92% | In-flight oxygen required (2 or 4 L/min) |
| Already receiving long-term oxygen therapy | Increase flow rate |

* Risk factor: $FEV_1 < 50\%$ predicted, lung cancer, respiratory muscle weakness and other restrictive ventilatory disorders, within 6 weeks of hospital discharge.

# CHAPTER 12

# Exacerbations

*Graeme P. Currie*

Aberdeen Royal Infirmary, Aberdeen, UK

### OVERVIEW

- Exacerbations are important events in the natural history of chronic obstructive pulmonary disease (COPD) and are associated with a more rapid decline in lung function and health status.
- Treat exacerbations of COPD promptly; doing so confers short-, medium- and long-term benefit.
- Inhaled bronchodilators form the mainstay of treatment.
- Give short courses of oral corticosteroids in most exacerbations affecting daily activities.
- Antibiotics are most effective when there is a combination of increased breathlessness and increased sputum volume and purulence.
- If admitted to hospital, aim for oxygen saturation between 88% and 92% in those with a history of type 2 (hypercapnic) respiratory failure; aim for oxygen saturations of 94–98% in others.
- Non-invasive ventilation has revolutionised the management of hypercapnic exacerbations.
- Aminophylline has a limited role in the management of exacerbations of COPD.
- Following an exacerbation, explore non-pharmacological and pharmacological strategies based around prevention.
- Hospital admission and discharge care bundles may lead to better outcomes.

## Definition

An exacerbation of chronic obstructive pulmonary disease (COPD) can be defined as a sustained worsening of respiratory symptoms that is acute in onset and usually requires a patient to seek medical help or alter medication. The deterioration must also be more severe than the usual variation experienced by the individual on a daily basis. Variations in the definition of an exacerbation exist from country to country and guideline to guideline (although many similarities are shared); these are often tailored further in the context of randomised clinical trials as they frequently represent important – and often primary – endpoints.

While important events in the natural history of COPD, exacerbations (and their frequency) play a pivotal role in the characterisation of patients in the Global Initiative for Chronic Obstructive Lung Disease (GOLD) guidelines which in turn help guide appropriate management.

## Mechanism

Airway neutrophils, in addition to an array of local and systemic inflammatory mediators, are increased during exacerbations of COPD (Figure 12.1). A minority of exacerbations are associated with increased airway eosinophils. The overwhelming inflammatory cell influx leads to airflow obstruction, lung hyperinflation, ventilation/perfusion mismatch and increased oxygen demands and pulmonary artery pressure.

The breathlessness that occurs during an acute exacerbation is partly due to the consequences of dynamic hyperinflation (associated with increased residual volume and reduction in inspiratory capacity). This is in response to airway obstruction and places the lungs at a mechanical disadvantage. Markers of lung hyperinflation generally improve as recovery takes place.

## Clinical features

Exacerbations are typically characterised by a combination of increased:
- breathlessness
- cough
- sputum volume
- sputum purulence
- wheeze
- chest tightness.

Other common clinical features include malaise, reduction in exercise tolerance, tachypnoea, tachycardia, peripheral oedema, accessory muscle use, confusion and cyanosis. Many other (often co-existing) cardiorespiratory disorders can also cause some of these features and are included in the differential diagnosis (Box 12.1).

*ABC of COPD*, Third Edition. Edited by Graeme P. Currie.
© 2017 John Wiley & Sons Ltd. Published 2017 by John Wiley & Sons Ltd.

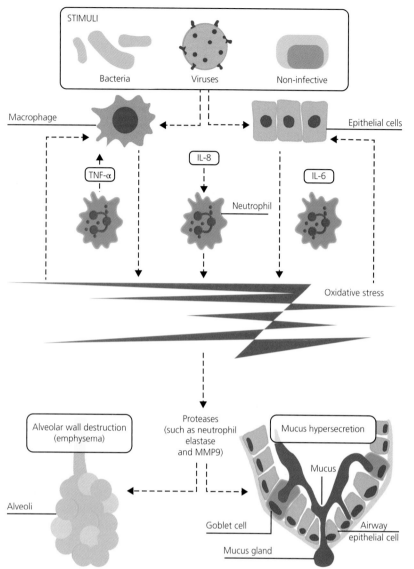

**Figure 12.1** Mechanism for acute exacerbations in COPD. Triggers of COPD exacerbations include infectious agents such as bacteria and viruses and non-infectious agents such as air pollution. These stimuli activate airway epithelial cells and macrophages to release inflammatory cytokines including tumor necrosis factor-α (TNF-α), interleukin (IL)-8 and IL-6. These cytokines lead to neutrophil recruitment and the release of reactive oxidant species and proteases from activated neutrophils, which magnify the inflammatory process. Reproduced with permission from Aaron S. *BMJ* 2014; **349**: g5237.

---

Box 12.1 **Differential diagnosis of an exacerbation of COPD.**

- Exacerbation of asthma
- Bronchopneumonia
- Pulmonary embolism
- Pleural effusion
- Lung cancer
- Bronchiectasis
- Pneumothorax
- Upper airway obstruction
- Pulmonary oedema
- Cardiac arrhythmia, e.g. atrial fibrillation with uncontrolled ventricular response
- Idiopathic pulmonary fibrosis

---

The time for lung function to recover after a straightforward exacerbation is approximately 7–10 days, although symptoms typically take several days longer to return to baseline levels. Exacerbations can manifest within a day but a similar proportion of individuals may have a more gradual onset of symptoms over several days. Sudden exacerbations have been associated with increased respiratory symptoms but shorter recovery times.

## Aetiology

Exacerbations of COPD are complex events and are due to the interplay between the host and bacteria, viruses and environmental pollutants (Box 12.2). Viruses are thought to be implicated in causing around 50% of all exacerbations, with rhinoviruses and respiratory syncytial virus being the most commonly implicated. Viruses may also damage the airway epithelium and predispose to bacterial infection, while in combination, they may exert a synergistic inflammatory effect. Bacteria can frequently be found in the sputum of clinically stable patients, and it is not clear whether exacerbations are caused by mutation of existing bacteria

- Viruses
  - Rhinovirus
  - Respiratory syncytial virus
  - Influenza
  - Parainfluenza
  - Coronavirus
  - Adenovirus
- Bacteria
  - *Haemophilus influenzae*
  - *Streptococcus pneumoniae*
  - *Haemophilus parainfluenzae*
  - *Moraxella catarrhalis*
  - *Staphylococcus aureus*
  - *Pseudomonas aeruginosa*
  - Gram-negative bacilli
- Other organisms
  - *Chlamydia pneumoniae*
  - *Mycoplasma pneumoniae*
- Environmental pollutants
  - Ozone ($O_3$)
  - Sulphur dioxide ($SO_2$)
  - Nitrogen dioxide ($NO_2$)
  - Diesel exhaust fumes
- Cigarette smoke

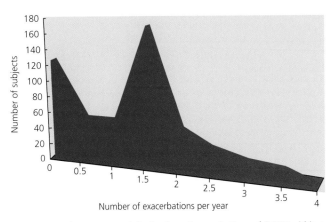

**Figure 12.2** The non-normal distribution of exacerbations of COPD within a population. Source: Scott S, Walker P, Calverley PMA. COPD exacerbations: prevention. *Thorax* 2006; **61**: 440–447. Reproduced with permission of BMJ Publishing Group Ltd.

Box 12.3 **Investigations usually required in patients admitted to hospital.**

- Full blood count
- Biochemistry and glucose
- Theophylline concentration (in patients using a theophylline preparation)
- Arterial blood gas (documenting the amount of oxygen given and by what delivery device)
- Electrocardiograph
- Chest X-ray
- Blood cultures in febrile patients
- Sputum microscopy, culture and sensitivity

or the acquisition of new bacterial strains. In up to a third of severe exacerbations, a specific cause is not identified.

## Impact

Exacerbations of COPD vary widely from mild episodes which can easily be managed at home to life-threatening events necessitating ventilatory support and a prolonged hospital stay. As a consequence, they have wide-reaching financial implications for secondary care providers and are likely to be partly responsible for high hospital and intensive care bed occupancy rates. With the ever-increasing aged population, it is likely that the numbers of exacerbations treated both in the community and within hospitals will continue to rise. Data relating to inpatient mortality from COPD are variable, with estimates ranging between 4% and 30%; the vast majority of acute episodes treated within the community do not result in death. Mortality within a few years of a severe exacerbation may even be as high as 50%.

Patients with a history of frequent exacerbations have an accelerated decline in lung function and health status, impaired quality of life and restriction of daily living activities. This in turn increases the likelihood of a patient becoming housebound. Individuals with more advanced disease usually experience more exacerbations, although there is fairly wide interindividual variation. Some individuals appear susceptible to a greater exacerbation frequency and more rapid decline in lung function than others, while the frequency of exacerbations is linked to mortality (Figure 12.2).

## Investigations

If admitted to hospital, investigate patients as shown in Box 12.3.

## Management

### Oxygen

Administration of oxygen is vital in all patients with respiratory failure to reduce breathlessness and prevent major organ and tissue hypoxaemia (see Chapter 11 for a more detailed description). In patients with type 2 respiratory failure, give controlled oxygen (24% or 28%) through a Venturi system to keep the oxygen saturation at 88–92%. In individuals with type 1 respiratory failure, titrate the oxygen concentration upwards to achieve a target saturation range of 94–98%. After giving oxygen for 30 minutes to 1 hour, recheck arterial blood gas levels, especially in those with type 2 respiratory failure (Table 12.1). This allows detection of a rise in carbon dioxide level or fall in pH due to loss of hypoxic drive. Deteriorating oxygen saturation or increasing breathlessness in a patient with previously stable hypoxaemia should also prompt repeat arterial blood gas measurements.

**Table 12.1** Arterial blood gas features of type 1 and type 2 respiratory failure.

| Parameter | Normal healthy range | Type 1 respiratory failure | Type 2 respiratory failure |
|---|---|---|---|
| $pO_2$ | 10–12 kPa | ↓ (<8 kPa) | ↓ (<8 kPa) |
| $pCO_2$ | 4.6–6 kPa | ↔ or ↓ | ↑ |
| $HCO_3$ | 23–27 mmol/L | ↔ | ↑ or ↔ |
| pH | 7.35–7.45 | ↔ or ↑ | ↔ or ↓ |

↑, increase; ↓, decrease; ↔, no change.

## Bronchodilators

Short-acting bronchodilators ($\beta_2$-agonists and anticholinergics) form the mainstay of treatment in exacerbations as they reduce symptoms and improve lung function. $\beta_2$-agonists (such as salbutamol) increase the concentrations of cyclic adenosine monophosphate (cAMP) and stimulate $\beta_2$-adrenoceptors, producing smooth muscle relaxation and bronchodilation, while anticholinergics (such as ipratropium) exert bronchodilator effects predominantly by inhibition at muscarinic receptors. Salbutamol has an onset of action within 5 minutes, while ipratropium takes effect at 10–15 minutes. Although there are few data supporting any additional benefit in acute exacerbations, both classes of short-acting bronchodilators are often given together.

Short-acting bronchodilators can successfully be given by a metered dose inhaler plus spacer or nebuliser with similar efficacy. However, nebulisers (with a mouthpiece or facemask) are independent of patient effort and more convenient than hand-held devices in emergency departments or busy ward settings. In patients with hypercapnia or respiratory acidosis, administer nebulised bronchodilators driven by compressed air and give supplemental oxygen via a nasal cannula (Figure 12.3).

## Corticosteroids

Over the years, studies have generally shown that systemic corticosteroids are of benefit in exacerbations of COPD. The mechanism by which they exert effects is uncertain, although they may reduce airway oedema and inflammation, in addition to attenuating the systemic inflammatory response. Some data have shown that using biomarkers (such as peripheral blood eosinophils) may help in determining preferential responses to oral corticosteroids.

In a Cochrane review across 16 studies, use of systemic corticosteroids (oral or intravenous) compared to placebo in COPD exacerbations resulted in reduced chances of treatment failure, relapse, length of hospital stay and earlier improvement in lung function and symptoms. No difference was found between oral versus intravenous administration.

In the absence of major contraindications, give oral corticosteroids to all patients with an exacerbation of COPD (Figure 12.4). In severely ill patients or in those who are unable to swallow, 100–200 mg of intravenous hydrocortisone 8–12 hourly is a suitable alternative. In most exacerbations, guidelines recommend 30–40 mg of prednisolone for between 7 and 14 days; little further benefit is found in longer dosing regimes and these should generally be avoided. However, a Cochrane review of eight studies did demonstrate that shorter courses (lasting 5 days) were likely to be as effective as longer (10–14 days) courses. In patients using oral corticosteroids for <3 weeks, it is not usually necessary to taper the dose downwards before discontinuation.

## Antibiotics

Individuals with COPD have relatively high concentrations of bacteria in their airways during both exacerbations and periods of clinical stability, although the overall benefits of antibiotics remain contentious. Injudicious antibiotic use may be implicated in the emergence of resistant strains of bacteria and enteric infections

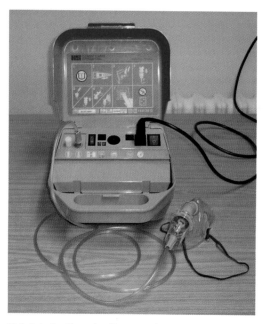

**Figure 12.3** Nebulised bronchodilators are frequently given during an exacerbation of COPD.

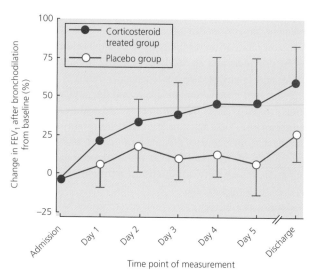

**Figure 12.4** Difference in forced expiratory volume in 1 second ($FEV_1$) with oral corticosteroids compared to placebo in patients admitted with an exacerbation of COPD. Source: Davies L, Angus R, Calverley P. Oral corticosteroids in patients admitted to hospital with exacerbations of chronic obstructive pulmonary disease: a prospective randomised controlled trial. *Lancet* 1999; **354**: 456–460. Reproduced with permission of Elsevier.

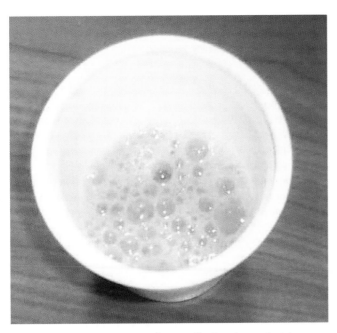

**Figure 12.5** Antibiotics are generally most effective when patients have increased breathlessness along with greater sputum volume and purulence.

such as *Clostridium difficile*, while many exacerbations are caused by viruses and pollutants. In a Cochrane review across 16 trials in patients with COPD exacerbations, beneficial effects of antibiotics were inconsistent. For example, large and consistent beneficial effects were found in patients admitted to intensive care, although antibiotics had no statistically significant effect on mortality and length of hospital stay in all other patients admitted to hospital.

Most guidelines suggest that antibiotics are most effective when patients have more severe exacerbations (especially with increased breathlessness) along with increased sputum volume and purulence (Figure 12.5). Patients with exacerbations without purulent sputum do not necessarily need antibiotics unless there is consolidation on chest X-ray or clinical features of pneumonia. When sputum has been sent for culture, the necessity and type of antibiotics should be checked against results once available.

The oral route is preferred unless the patient is vomiting, severely unwell or unable to swallow. Tailor the antibiotic to local sensitivities and guidance; amoxicillin for 5 days (or clarithromycin or doxycycline in penicillin-allergic patients) is a reasonable first-line choice in those with a mild to moderate exacerbation. In a severe exacerbation, consider intravenous and then oral co-trimoxazole (or clarithromycin). In some patients with advanced and end-stage disease, *Pseudomonas aeruginosa* can often be cultured, and if so, consider oral or intravenous antipseudomonal antibiotics.

## Aminophylline

Aminophylline has historically been used in exacerbations of COPD, despite a paucity of data demonstrating any major benefit. When compared to placebo, aminophylline has only limited (if any) effect upon symptoms, lung function and length of hospital stay in non-acidotic patients. Moreover, its use is associated with adverse

effects such as nausea, vomiting and tachyarrythmias. The routine addition of aminophylline in most exacerbations of COPD is therefore not warranted. Increasing evidence suggests that even at low doses, theophylline activates histone deacetylases (thereby attenuating the effects of activated proinflammatory mechanisms), although within the context of an exacerbation, the significance (if any) of this is uncertain.

Guidelines therefore suggest that aminophylline in conjunction with standard therapy should *only* be considered in patients with moderate-to-severe exacerbations or those not responding to nebulised bronchodilators and other treatments. However, with the widespread use of non-invasive ventilation (NIV), aminophylline now plays a minor role (if any). In patients not using an oral theophylline preparation, give a loading dose of 5 mg/kg over at least 20 minutes with cardiac monitoring with subsequent maintenance infusion of 0.5 mg/kg/h. In patients already using a theophylline preparation, omit the loading dose and check plasma level ideally prior to commencement of a maintenance infusion of 0.5 mg/kg/h. Measure daily plasma theophylline levels and alter the infusion rate to maintain a concentration of between 10 and 20 mg/L (55–110 µmol/L).

### Non-invasive ventilation

Non-invasive ventilation has revolutionised the management of hypercapnic respiratory failure due to COPD and is discussed in Chapter 13.

## General hospital care

Consider measures to prevent venous thromboembolism with low molecular weight heparin in all patients admitted with an exacerbation of COPD. Attend to hydration and nutritional needs in those with more severe exacerbations and advanced disease. Some patients may even benefit from nasogastric feeding, especially when too breathless to eat or when NIV is used for prolonged time periods. Intravenous magnesium is advocated in exacerbations of asthma, but is of no known benefit in COPD. It should therefore not be given.

Many patients also have important co-morbidities – for example, ischaemic heart disease, left ventricular dysfunction and diabetes mellitus – which must not be overlooked. Ensure routine drugs for other medical conditions are prescribed along with usual inhaled long-acting bronchodilators and corticosteroids.

Try to arrange early pulmonary rehabilitation and physiotherapy as soon after an exacerbation as possible; doing so may result in improvements in exercise capacity and overall health status. When recovering from an exacerbation, some patients may benefit from review by physiotherapists, occupational therapists and/or members of the social service team. Physiotherapists may be able to provide advice on breathlessness, panic and anxiety management, energy conservation techniques and walking aids, while occupational therapists and social service team members can offer practical solutions when problems exist with daily living activities.

### Assisted hospital discharge

Any intervention which successfully hastens a patient's recovery and discharge from hospital can be potentially useful in the overall management of an exacerbation. In recent years, 'assisted hospital

Box 12.4 **Relative contraindications to assisted hospital discharge in patients with an exacerbation of COPD.**

- Acute onset
- Confusion
- Worsening peripheral oedema
- Uncertain diagnosis
- Poor performance status
- Concomitant unstable medical disorders
- New chest X-ray abnormalities
- Acidosis or marked hypoxia or hypercapnia
- Adverse social conditions

discharge' or 'hospital at home' schemes have been developed. These allow patients with non-severe exacerbations to be discharged fairly immediately back into the community (after initial assessment in hospital) with appropriate nursing and medical back-up. Apart from providing patients with a package of care, this practice also facilitates the identification of a deterioration in clinical condition and readmission to hospital if necessary. Studies have shown that hospital readmission and mortality rates are not significantly different when assisted discharge schemes are compared to standard inpatient care. Moreover, such schemes may lead to financial savings along with increased availability of inpatient beds. Not all patients admitted with an exacerbation of COPD are suitable for assisted discharge, and relative contraindications are highlighted in Box 12.4.

## Monitoring in hospital

Clinical assessment and routine observations are useful in assessing the rate of recovery from an exacerbation. Frequent arterial blood gas measurements are also required to monitor patients with decompensated respiratory acidosis – in some patients requiring prolonged NIV, an arterial line may be useful. Daily recordings of peak expiratory flow rates are less useful, unless the patient has reversible obstructive lung disease. It can be useful to perform spirometry prior to discharge as this helps confirm the diagnosis (in patients who have not previously had it performed), provides information regarding the severity of airflow obstruction and enables progress to be assessed at subsequent outpatient follow-up.

## Care bundles

In recent years there has been increasing interest in the use of 'care bundles' when dealing with patients with COPD exacerbations. These comprise a series of structured and standardised steps (which must be followed) that patients receive when admitted or discharged from hospital and incorporate different aspects of management. Some evidence exists that implementation of such care bundles are associated with better outcomes and patient satisfaction, although further work is needed.

Examples of criteria which might be included in an admission care bundle are:

- establishing a correct diagnosis of an exacerbation of COPD (for example, with the help of a chest X-ray performed within a predefined period of time plus a note of historical spirometry)

- assessing oxygenation and prescribing a target saturation range within 1 hour of admission
- recognising and responding to respiratory acidosis and hypercapnia
- initiating correct treatment within a set time from admission
- arranging review by a respiratory specialist within 24 hours of admission.

Examples of features which might appear on a discharge care bundle include:

- assessing and correcting inhaler technique
- ensuring patients receive appropriate inhaled drugs
- provision of a written self-management plan
- assessing smoking status and advising on how to quit
- offering pulmonary rehabilitation and arranging where appropriate
- telephone follow-up within several days of discharge.

## Outpatient follow-up

Arrange early follow-up following hospital discharge (e.g. within 3 weeks), in either the community or secondary care, as this may help prevent readmission. This also gives an opportunity to explore strategies to prevent a further exacerbation and provide education, check inhaler technique, alter inhaled treatment if required, check oxygen saturation and arterial blood gases where necessary and reassess smoking status.

It should also be made clear to patients that exacerbations should be promptly treated in the future; doing so results in quicker recovery and leads to better outcomes than if a delay occurs. Patients who frequently fail to promptly report or recognise worsening symptoms have a greater risk of being admitted to hospital and generally have a poorer quality of life.

## Frequent exacerbations

It is well established that many patients with COPD have frequent exacerbations necessitating repeated hospital admissions. This is especially the case in individuals with hypercapnic respiratory failure who have had treatment with NIV. Indeed, within a year after hospital discharge, it is likely that the majority of these patients will be readmitted to hospital and require further NIV, with as many as half dying.

## Prevention of exacerbations

Consider ways to prevent an exacerbation in all patients admitted with such an event. Many non-pharmacological and pharmacological strategies reduce the frequency of exacerbations of COPD. Examples of these include early pulmonary rehabilitation, lung volume reduction surgery, long-term oxygen, long-acting bronchodilators, inhaled corticosteroids, macrolides and mucolytics, details of which are discussed in separate chapters.

## Further reading

Aaron SD, Donaldson GC, Whitmore GA, Hurst JR, Ramsay T, Wedzicha JA. Time course and pattern of COPD exacerbation onset. *Thorax* 2012; **67**: 238–243.

Barr RG, Rowe BH, Camargo CA Jr. Methylxanthines for exacerbations of chronic obstructive pulmonary disease. *Cochrane Database of Systematic Reviews* 2003; **2**: CD002168.

Chu CM, Chan VL, Lin AWN, Wong IWY, Leung WS, Lai CKW. Readmission rates and life-threatening events in COPD survivors treated with non-invasive ventilation for hypercapnic respiratory failure. *Thorax* 2004; **59**: 1020–1025.

Man WD, Polkey MI, Donaldson N, Gray BJ, Moxham J. Community pulmonary rehabilitation after hospitalisation for acute exacerbations of chronic obstructive pulmonary disease: randomised controlled study. *BMJ* 2004; **329**: 1209.

McCrory DC, Brown CD. Anticholinergic bronchodilators versus beta2- sympathomimetic agents for acute exacerbations of chronic obstructive pulmonary disease. *Cochrane Database of Systematic Reviews* 2002; **3**: CD003900.

Ospina MB, Mrklas K, Deuchar L, Rowe BH, Leigh R, Bhutani M, Stickland MK. A systematic review of the effectiveness of discharge care bundles for patients with COPD. *Thorax* 2016; **72**: 31–39.

Puhan MA, Gimeno-Santos E, Scharplatz M et al. Pulmonary rehabilitation following exacerbations of chronic obstructive pulmonary disease. *Cochrane Database of Systematic Reviews* 2011; **10**: CD005305.

Quon BS, Gan WQ, Sin DD. Contemporary management of acute exacerbations of COPD: a systematic review and meta-analysis. *Chest* 2008; **133**: 756–766.

Rodríguez-Roisin R. COPD exacerbations: management. *Thorax* 2006; **61**: 535–544.

Seemungal TA, Donaldson GC, Bhowmik A, Jeffries DJ, Wedzicha JA. Time course and recovery of exacerbations in patients with chronic obstructive pulmonary disease. *American Journal of Respiratory and Critical Care Medicine* 2000; **161**: 1608–1613.

Vollenweider DJ, Jarrett H, Steurer-Stey CA, Garcia-Aymerich J, Puhan MA. Antibiotics for exacerbations of chronic obstructive pulmonary disease. *Cochrane Database of Systematic Reviews* 2012; **12**: CD010257.

Walters JAE, Tan DJ, White CJ, Gibson PG, Wood-Baker R, Walters EH. Systemic corticosteroids for acute exacerbations of chronic obstructive pulmonary disease. *Cochrane Database of Systematic Reviews* 2014; **9**: CD001288.

Walters JAE, Tan DJ, White CJ, Wood-Baker R. Different durations of corticosteroid therapy for exacerbations of chronic obstructive pulmonary disease. *Cochrane Database of Systematic Reviews* 2014; **12**: CD006897.

Wilkinson TMA, Donaldson GC, Hurst JR, Seemungal TAR, Wedzicha JA. Early therapy improves outcomes of exacerbations of chronic obstructive pulmonary disease. *American Journal of Respiratory and Critical Care Medicine* 2004; **168**: 1298–1303.

# CHAPTER 13

# Ventilatory Support

*Paul K. Plant*[1], *Stephen Stott*[2] *and Graeme P. Currie*[2]

[1]North Cumbria University Hospital NHS Trust, Carlisle, UK
[2]Aberdeen Royal Infirmary, Aberdeen, UK

## OVERVIEW

In exacerbations of chronic obstructive pulmonary disease (COPD):

- non-invasive ventilation (NIV) reduces mortality and the need for intubation in patients with a respiratory acidosis (pH <7.35 and $PaCO_2 > 6\,kPa$)

- consider NIV within 1 hour of hospital arrival in all patients who have a persisting respiratory acidosis despite maximum medical therapy

- ensure NIV is initiated only by trained staff; monitoring should include respiratory rate, arterial blood gases, pulse oximetry, assessment of synchrony and compliance

- continue NIV until the underlying acute cause has resolved and pH returns to normal limits, or when it is no longer appropriate to administer

- NIV should be weaned gradually and not abruptly

- ensure all patients have a clear plan recorded and agreed upon in case of NIV failure

- domiciliary NIV plays a very limited role in managing patients with recurrent exacerbations

- consider invasive mechanical ventilation in patients who fail to improve with NIV.

Non-invasive ventilation (NIV) is the gold standard treatment for patients with acute exacerbations of chronic obstructive pulmonary disease (COPD) complicated by decompensated (or partially compensated) type 2 respiratory failure (defined as pH <7.35 and $PaCO_2 > 6\,kPa$) despite immediate medical therapy. It is safe and effective in a variety of settings, recommended by the National Institute of Health and Care Excellence (NICE), and well established within all national and international guidelines. Patients with acute exacerbations of COPD should ideally only be admitted to facilities where NIV is readily available. To help deliver an effective NIV service, ensure a regularly updated written protocol is available (and updated), and that a named clinical lead plus cohort of dedicated, suitably trained and enthusiastic multidisciplinary team members are empowerd. Incorporate audit of outcomes and reviews of practice on a regular (preferably annual) basis.

## Why is non-invasive ventilation useful?

When receiving NIV, patients are able to communicate, eat, drink, undergo physiotherapy and receive nebulised and oral medication more easily than with other forms of ventilation (Figure 13.1).

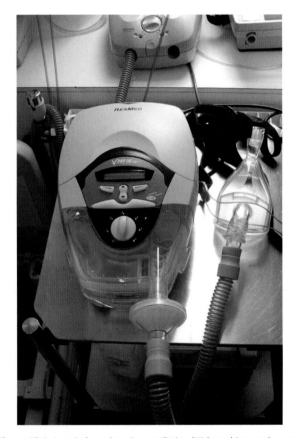

**Figure 13.1** A typical non-invasive ventilation (NIV) machine can be easily used at the patient's bedside.

---

*ABC of COPD*, Third Edition. Edited by Graeme P. Currie.
© 2017 John Wiley & Sons Ltd. Published 2017 by John Wiley & Sons Ltd.

NIV provides many other advantages over invasive mechanical ventilation (IMV) (Box 13.1).

---

Box 13.1 **Advantages of NIV over invasive mechanical ventilation.**

- Patients can eat and drink
- Patients can communicate and make decisions about management
- Patients maintain a physiological cough
- Physiological warming and humidification occur
- No sedatives required
- Reduced risk of ventilator-associated pneumonia
- Less expensive
- Less wasteful of resources
- Allows intermittent use (which facilitates weaning)
- Endotracheal intubation remains an option

---

## Which patients with COPD should receive non-invasive ventilation?

Within hospitals, local guidelines and criteria for the initiation of NIV in COPD exacerbations should be widely available and known to all staff responsible for the care of such patients. In particular, consider NIV in the following circumstances.

- Persisting decompensated respiratory acidosis (within 60 minutes of arriving in hospital) despite initial aggressive therapy, including use of controlled oxygen
- As a therapeutic trial prior to proceeding to IMV
- Weaning from IMV
- As an adjunct to palliation of symptoms

Prior to starting NIV, decide and document whether the patient is a suitable candidate for IMV and consider whether relative contraindications to NIV exist. Caution is advised in commencing NIV in moribund patients with multiorgan failure in whom intubation (at one end of the extreme) or a palliative approach (at the other end) might be far more appropriate and pragmatic initial strategies. However, for patients who are 'not for intubation', have impaired consciousness and/or severe respiratory acidosis, NIV can still be administered with good effect. In such patients, a nasal or oropharyngeal airway may be required. The views of the patient and family as to whether they would wish further respiratory support if NIV proves unsuccessful should also be taken into account. Clearly document any escalation plan (or otherwise) within the medical and nursing notes. Although NIV can be used in individuals with exacerbations of COPD with radiological evidence of pneumonia, outcomes are generally less favourable (Box 13.2).

---

Box 13.2 **Relative contraindications to NIV; none of these are absolute and the clinical context needs to be considered.**

- Confusion/agitation
- Inability to maintain airway
- Reduced Glasgow Coma Scale
- Haemodynamic instability

- Vomiting
- Copious respiratory secretions and risk of aspiration
- Facial burns/surgery/trauma
- Severe hypoxia
- Untreated pneumothorax
- Severe pneumonia/sepsis
- Fixed upper airway obstruction
- Bowel obstruction
- Bronchopleural fistula

---

## How non-invasive ventilation works

A close-fitting face or nose mask connected to a portable ventilator by plastic tubing provides a non-invasive method of respiratory support (mechanically assisted or mechanically generated breaths) to the spontaneously breathing patient. NIV provides a bi-level form of respiratory support. Ventilation is provided by inspiratory positive airways pressure (IPAP), which is usually titrated from 10 to between 15 and 20 $cmH_2O$. This helps to offload tiring respiratory muscles and reduce the work of breathing, improve alveolar ventilation and oxygenation and increase $CO_2$ elimination.

During expiration, the expiratory positive airway pressure (EPAP) helps 'splint open' the airway and flush $CO_2$ from the mask. It also reduces the work of breathing by overcoming intrinsic positive end expiratory pressure, thereby reducing atelectasis and increasing end tidal volume; usual pressures are between 4 and 6 $cmH_2O$.

Oxygen is usually introduced either through a port in the facemask or through a channel found more proximally in the ventilator system. The exact fraction of inspired oxygen delivered to the patient is usually unknown and oxygen entrainment should be titrated against pulse oximetry. Humidification is rarely required.

## Outcomes of non-invasive ventilation

Many studies with differing endpoints – such as mortality, need for intubation, arterial blood gas values and cost-effectiveness – have consistently shown significant benefits with NIV over and above conventional medical treatment alone. For example, a meta-analysis of eight randomised controlled trials evaluated effects of NIV in patients admitted with an exacerbation of COPD with $pCO_2 > 6$ kPa. This study demonstrated that compared to standard treatment alone, the use of concomitant NIV was associated with:

- lower mortality
- reduced need for intubation
- reduced likelihood of treatment failure
- lower complication rates
- improvements at 1 hour in pH, $pCO_2$ and respiratory rate
- shorter hospital stays.

## Setting

Non-invasive ventilation can be successfully used in the ward setting, emergency department and high-dependency and intensive care units (ICU). The setting where NIV is provided is less important than the availability of suitably trained and experienced staff who can initiate treatment, monitor progress and troubleshoot. There is no lower limit of pH at which NIV becomes inappropriate and it can be used alongside other measures (such as inotropes) to support other failing organs.

For patients with COPD, there is little to guide ventilator selection other than familiarity, ease of use, cost and local preference. If NIV is used for hypoxic respiratory failure, the ventilator unit needs an intrinsic blender to ensure that high fractions of inspired oxygen can be delivered. ICU ventilators are often difficult to use non-invasively as they are poorly leak tolerant and alarm readily.

## How to use non-invasive ventilation

Provided the clinical condition permits, show the patient the ventilator, facemask and tubing; an appropriately sized facemask (sizing rings are usually provided by the manufacturer) should then be chosen. Nasal masks may also be used and are comfortable for long-term use, but require the patient to breathe through their nose. However, most patients with COPD breathe through their mouth and full facemasks are preferable (Figure 13.2). It is useful if the mask is first placed on the patient for a few minutes prior to securing it with straps. Set oxygen at an initial appropriate flow rate (typically 1–2 L/min) and adjust to maintain $SpO_2$ between 88% and 92%.

Set the IPAP and EPAP at fairly low pressures such as 10 and 4 cmH$_2$O respectively. The inspiratory pressure can then be titrated up in 5 cmH$_2$O increments (approximately every 10 minutes) to 15–20 cmH$_2$O or to the maximum pressure comfortably tolerated. Depending on the type of ventilator, other parameters such as the sensitivity of inspiratory and expiratory triggers and maximum inspiratory and expiratory times may be set. Adjustments to these may be necessary to maximise synchrony between the ventilator and the efforts of the patient. Once started, patient comfort, breathing synchrony and compliance are key factors for success with NIV. In some individuals with shallow breathing or low respiratory rates, it may be necessary to programme the NIV machine to deliver a minimum number of breaths per minute. In patients with co-existing COPD and obstructive sleep apnoea/hypopnoea syndrome, higher pressures, for example EPAP 10 cmH$_2$O and IPAP 20–25 cmH$_2$O, may be required. For intubated patients, NIV should be used as part of the weaning strategy. Doing so may be associated with shorter ICU stays, better survival and earlier weaning.

## Monitoring non-invasive ventilation

Irrespective of $PaO_2$ or $PaCO_2$, the pH is a reliable marker of severity in exacerbations of COPD, and is closely linked to mortality and the need for intubation. In addition to regular recording of pulse, blood pressure and respiratory rate, the oxygen saturation should be monitored and number of hours of NIV use documented. Check arterial blood gases 1 hour after starting NIV; an improvement in pH and pCO$_2$ and reduction in respiratory rate are good prognostic signs (Figure 13.3). If no improvement occurs, the mask should be checked for leaks, all tubing and connections checked for problems, the ventilator checked for synchrony with the patient's respiratory effort and consideration given to adjusting ventilator settings (e.g. increasing IPAP or EPAP, or altering the oxygen flow rate). Recheck blood gases 4–6 hours after NIV initiation (or earlier in the event of a clinical deterioration) and within 1 hour of a change in ventilator setting. In general, try to make a decision to proceed to IMV (or otherwise) within 4 hours of initiation of NIV.

Continue NIV until it is no longer appropriate (due to continual deterioration) or the underlying acute cause and acidosis has resolved (typically for 3–4 days, although sometimes only 24 hours (or less) of treatment is required). Do not discontinue NIV as soon as the pH first normalises. Weaning from NIV is rarely a problem, as patients normally 'auto wean' by progressively decreasing their use automatically. Treatment reduction should affect day

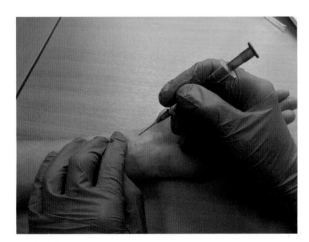

**Figure 13.3** Frequent monitoring of arterial blood gases is required in patients using NIV. This should be performed prior to starting NIV and 1 and 4–6 hours afterwards; it should also be checked within an hour of changing settings. An arterial line is often a more convenient way by which to obtain regular blood gas measurements, especially if it is felt likely that NIV will be required for a prolonged period of time.

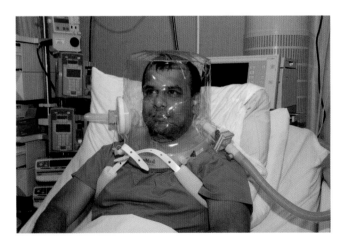

**Figure 13.2** An NIV hood can be used in patients intolerant of either a full face or nasal mask.

time ventilation periods initially. After withdrawal of ventilatory support during the day, a further night of NIV is often recommended/required.

## Other measures

In patients commenced on NIV, maximal medical therapy such as nebulised bronchodilators, corticosteroids and antibiotics should be continued. Give nebulised bronchodilators during 'NIV-free' periods when possible, as NIV impairs aerosol formation and lung delivery. Try to avoid sedative drugs such as benzodiazepines and opiates, which may affect upper airway tone/patency; if these drugs are used prior to admission, pharmacological reversal may be required if the respiratory rate or Glasgow Coma Scale is low. However, if patients are particularly agitated while receiving NIV, consider intravenous morphine (such as 2.5–5 mg), possibly with a short-acting benzodiazepine such as midazolam. This may facilitate symptom relief and improve tolerance of NIV.

Keep patients adequately hydrated and ensure an adequate calorific intake is maintained (Figure 13.4). NIV can be used with a nasogastric tube in place; use a fine-bore tube to minimise mask leakage. It is not necessary to place a nasogastric tube simply because a patient is to receive NIV.

## Problems with non-invasive ventilation

The majority of patients tolerate NIV without significant problems. However, some patients experience difficulty in 'breathing with the machine'. The mask can be associated with problems such as claustrophobia, facial sores and persistent air leaks (Figure 13.5). Table 13.1 provides guidance on managing common problems. Patients who recover from an exacerbation treated with NIV are at high risk of a future exacerbation requiring NIV, and should be asked whether they would wish such ventilatory support in the future (record this in the case notes).

## Domiciliary non-invasive ventilation

Domiciliary NIV for stable COPD is generally not recommended. Unlike patients with neuromuscular disorders, adherence tends to be poorer following hospital discharge. Randomised controlled trials have failed to consistently show a definite survival advantage or quality of life, exercise tolerance or lung function improvement. However, in one study of 195 patients with stable COPD, $PaCO_2 > 7$ kPa, good exercise capacity and few exacerbations, a high-intensity approach to home NIV did confer mortality benefit after 1 year.

Regional variations in practice exist, but domiciliary NIV is sometimes adopted in carefully selected motivated patients with COPD requiring long-term oxygen therapy who frequently develop hypercapnia or acidosis on a regular basis (typically 3–4 exacerbations a year). Assess adherence and markers of usefulness (such as reduced number of hospital admission) on a regular basis.

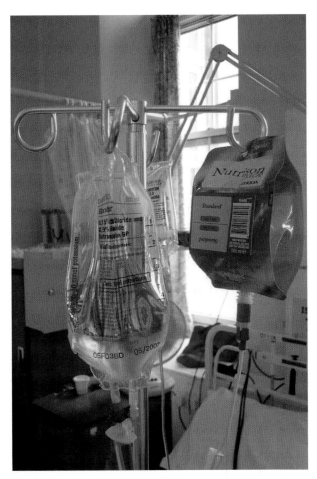

**Figure 13.4** Patients being treated with NIV can easily become dehydrated and undernourished; adequate hydration and nutrition should not be forgotten in overall management.

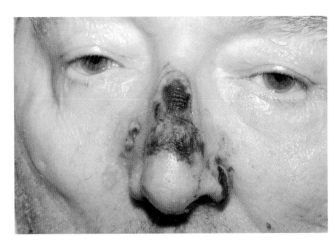

**Figure 13.5** Severe nasal bridge ulceration in a patient who required NIV for a prolonged period of time. As this problem may arise in up to 10% of patients receiving NIV, facemasks should not be tightened excessively. Reproduced with permission from Dr David Miller, Aberdeen Royal Infirmary, Aberdeen.

**Table 13.1** Problems associated with NIV and potential solutions.

| Problem | Possible solutions |
|---|---|
| Persistent hypoxia | Re-evaluate patient and optimise medical treatment |
| | Check compliance with ventilation and synchrony |
| | Check head position/airway |
| | Exclude pneumothorax |
| | Check oxygen tubing for leaks/blockages |
| | Increase oxygen flow rate |
| | Increase IPAP to a maximum of 25 cmH$_2$O |
| | Increase EPAP by small amounts |
| | Arrange intubation and ventilation |
| | Consider palliation (if NIV is the 'ceiling of treatment') |
| Persisting hypercapnia/respiratory acidosis | Re-evaluate patient and optimise medical treatment |
| | Check compliance with ventilation and synchrony |
| | Check head position/airway |
| | Exclude pneumothorax |
| | Avoid sedating drugs |
| | Increase IPAP to a maximum of 25 cmH$_2$O |
| | Reduce oxygen flow if saturation >88–92% |
| | Increase back-up rate if respiratory rate low |
| | Ensure expiratory port is patent |
| | Arrange intubation and ventilation |
| | Consider palliation (if NIV is the 'ceiling of treatment') |
| Respiratory alkalosis/hypocapnia | Reduce IPAP |
| | Reduce back-up respiratory rate |
| | Reduce hours of use |
| | Ensure serum potassium >4 mmol/L |
| Nasal/forehead ulceration | Loosen straps |
| | Apply dressing |
| | Longer 'rest periods' without NIV |
| | Consider full head mask/nasal plugs |
| Nasal congestion | Nasally inhaled corticosteroids |
| | Nasally inhaled decongestants (short-term use only) |
| | Change nasal mask to full facemask |
| | Humidification |
| Mask leak | Readjust straps and mask (may paradoxically require loosening) |
| | Change to a more suitably sized facemask |
| Claustrophobia | Consider different mask (nasal or full head mask) |
| | Allow patient to hold the mask in position |
| NIV dependence | More gradual discontinuation |
| | Distracting techniques while not using NIV |
| | Reassurance |
| Gastric distension | Reduce IPAP |
| | Reduce EPAP |
| | Insert a fine-bore nasogastric tube |
| Confusion/delirium | Monitor in high-dependency setting |
| | Minimise procedures and contacts |
| | Correct oxygen and carbon dioxide as soon as possible |
| | Consider other causes of confusion (such as alcohol or nicotine withdrawal) |
| | Consider sedative drugs (e.g. haloperidol) if persistently aggressive or agitated |

EPAP, expiratory positive airway pressure; IPAP, inspiratory positive airway pressure; NIV, non-invasive ventilation.

## Invasive mechanical ventilation

Invasive mechanical ventilation is the rescue treatment for patients with acute exacerbations of COPD when NIV has failed (or is failing) (Box 13.3); this can usually be determined by lack of improvement in PaCO$_2$, pH, respiratory rate and conscious level.

Outcomes of patients who need IMV are worse than those who do not, although 70% of these patients will be able to be weaned from a ventilator and 30% will survive to 1 year. Because of these survival statistics, IMV should not be denied to patients who fail to progress with NIV as careful case selection will increase weaning and survival chances.

- Initial pH <7.25
- Glasgow Coma Score <11/15
- Tachypnoea
- Respiratory rate >35
- Asynchronous breathing pattern
- Edentulous
- Agitation
- Excessive air leak
- Excessive secretions
- Failure to improve within 2 hours of NIV
- Rapid shallow breathing index (RSBI) >105 (respiratory rate (breaths per min)/tidal volume (mL))

Recognising that NIV is failing is an important part of patient management and it is important to have a documented agreed plan prior to this stage; trying to have a meaningful discussion about treatment options with a patient *in extremis* is fruitless. The key to early decision making is review of the patient's progress in the first few hours after commencing NIV.

## Transfer to the intensive care unit

If NIV is failing and the patient plan includes tracheal intubation, then this is best done early and in the ICU. Complications of tracheal intubation rise when intubation is performed outwith the ICU setting. Some hospitals use checklists to help facilitate the optimum time for ICU referral and transfer.

The decision to intubate is largely based on clinician experience. Helpful clinical signs include deteriorating gas exchange despite medical management, imminent cardiorespiratory arrest, severe respiratory distress (as evidenced by tachypneoa, nasal flaring, accessory muscle recruitment, tracheal tug, recession of the suprasternal and intercostal spaces, pulsus paradoxus, diaphoresis) and altered level of consciousness.

## Ventilator strategies

The basic pathophysiology in exacerbations of COPD is the critical expiratory airflow limitation with consequent dynamic hyperinflation with increased work of breathing. These changes lead to cardiac impairment and worsening acidosis and hypoxia which further exacerbate respiratory muscle function dysfunction. Ventilatory strategies are aimed at improving the gas exchange abnormality, and identifying and preventing dynamic hyperinflation.

Initial settings should include low tidal volumes (6 mL/kg), a high inspiratory flow rate, a lengthened expiratory time to facilitate time for expiration and a minute ventilation that limits plateau (alveolar pressure) to <30 cm/$H_2O$. Even with these settings, air trapping can occur which can cause auto-positive end expiratory pressure (high pressure inside alveoli) which can lead to excessive work of breathing or even cardiovascular collapse. Immediately after intubation, particular attention should be paid to the ventilator waveforms which can aid early identification.

It is not necessary to achieve normal gas exchange and targets for oxygen saturations of 88–92% and carbon dioxide levels which relate to a normal pH are recommended. Permissive hypercapnia (allowing the partial pressure of carbon dioxide to be at a higher level than the normal range) will allow adjustment of body bicarbonate which will aid muscle function and reduce weaning time. Complications of IMV in exacerbations of COPD are shown in Table 13.2.

Sedation is an important part of IMV. Titration of the dose to a defined endpoint is recommended with systematic tapering of the dose or a daily sedation break. This is when all sedative drugs are stopped each day and restarted after an assessment of the readiness to wean from the ventilator has been carried. As soon as possible, patient-initiated breaths should be encouraged as this will shorten weaning time and preserve respiratory muscle strength. This is often facilitated by a pressure support ventilator mode where the ventilator aids the patient-initiated breath. Weaning of this support allows gradual improvement in respiratory muscle strength.

If weaning is prolonged (typically >10 days) then a tracheostomy may be considered (Figure 13.6). In this procedure (performed either percutaneously or via an open surgical approach) an opening is created in the front of the neck into the trachea. The tracheostomy tube is placed through this. Tracheostomy can reduce the work of breathing by decreasing tube resistance, aiding clearance of secretions and allowing cessation of sedating drugs. It may also allow normal diet to be resumed and allows patient interaction with relatives and caregivers. In some cases of exacerbations of COPD, weaning from IMV can be prolonged and particular attention needs to be paid to avoidance of hospital-acquired infections, improving nutrition and psychological support to both the patient and relatives.

**Table 13.2** Complications of invasive mechanical ventilation.

| Immediate | Medium term | Longer term |
|---|---|---|
| Barotrauma | Hospital-acquired pneumonia | Critical illness polyneuropathy |
| Pneumothorax | Malnutrition | Psychological issues |
| Pneumomediastinum | Pressure ulcers | Malnutrition |
| Auto-positive end expiratory pressure | Stress peptic ulceration | |
| Cardiovascular collapse | Alveolar damage from positive pressure ventilation | |
| Endotracheal tube blockage/displacement | Toxicity from high inspired concentrations of oxygen leading to alveolar damage | |
| Excessive secretions | | |

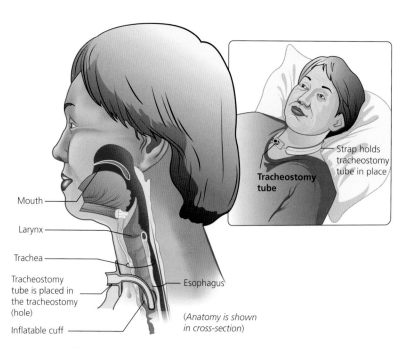

Mouth

Larynx

Trachea

Tracheostomy
tube is placed in
the tracheostomy
(hole)

Inflatable cuff

Esophagus

(*Anatomy is shown
in cross-section*)

**Tracheostomy
tube**

Strap holds
tracheostomy
tube in place

**Figure 13.6** Fashioning of a tracheostomy can help the weaning process; it can be left *in situ* for days, weeks or even months. It is usually well tolerated, although complications such as bleeding, infection, blockage, displacement or, less commonly, dysphagia, laryngeal damage, pneumothorax, tracheal stenosis, tracheomalacia or tracheo-oesophageal fistula may occur.

## Further reading

BTS/ICS guideline for the ventilatory management of acute hypercapnic respiratory failure in adults. *Thorax* 2016; **71**: ii1–ii35.

Kohnlein T, Windisch W, Kohler D et al. Non-invasive positive pressure ventilation for the treatment of severe stable chronic obstructive pulmonary disease: a prospective, multicentre, randomised, controlled clinical trial. *Lancet Respiratory Medicine* 2014; **2**: 698–705.

Lightowler JV, Wedzicha JA, Elliott, MW, Ram FSF. Non-invasive positive pressure ventilation to treat respiratory failure resulting from exacerbations of chronic obstructive pulmonary disease: Cochrane systematic review and meta-analysis. *BMJ* 2003; **326**: 185–190.

McLaughlin K, Thain G, Murray I, Currie GP. Ward based non-invasive ventilation for exacerbations of COPD: a real-life perspective. *Quarterly Journal of Medicine* 2010; **103**: 505–510.

Ocal S, Ortac Ersoy E, Ozturk O, Hayran M, Topeli A, Coplu L. Long-term outcome of chronic obstructive pulmonary disease patients with acute respiratory failure following intensive care unit discharge in Turkey. *Clinical Respiratory Journal* 2016; DOI:10.1111/crj.12450.

Plant PK, Owen JL, Elliott MW. One year period prevalence study of respiratory acidosis in acute exacerbations of COPD: implications for the provision of non-invasive ventilation and oxygen administration. *Thorax* 2000; **55**: 550–554.

Plant PK, Owen JL, Elliott MW. Non-invasive ventilation in acute exacerbations of chronic obstructive pulmonary disease: long-term survival and predictors of in-hospital outcome. *Thorax* 2001; **56**: 708–712.

Struik FM, Sprooten RT, Kerstjens HA et al. Nocturnal non-invasive ventilation in COPD patients with prolonged hypercapnia after ventilatory support for acute respiratory failure: a randomised, controlled, parallel-group study. *Thorax* 2014; **69**: 826–834.

# CHAPTER 14

# Primary Care

*Cathy Jackson*

School of Medicine, University of Central Lancashire, Preston, UK

---

> **OVERVIEW**
>
> - Chronic obstructive pulmonary disease (COPD) is extremely common in the UK but remains underdiagnosed.
> - Consider COPD as a diagnosis in all patients over the age of 35 who have a history of smoking.
> - The UK Quality Outcomes Framework (QOF) defines a set of clinical aims to guide primary care health teams.

Chronic obstructive pulmonary disease (COPD) is common in the UK and many other countries throughout the world where cigarette smoking is prevalent. According to the World Health Organization, approximately 65 million individuals worldwide are thought to have COPD although accurate figures are scarce. Ninety percent of deaths caused by COPD are likely to occur in low- to middle-income countries. It is estimated that in the UK, as many as 2 million individuals may have COPD which has not yet been diagnosed, and that tens of thousands of admissions for acute exacerbations each year occur in patients in whom a diagnosis of COPD has not yet been made. General practitioners (GPs) and primary healthcare teams are perhaps best placed to consider the diagnosis in all patients over the age of 35 who have a history of smoking. Consideration of the possibility of the disease in all smokers allows for screening, early and effective management and a 'teachable moment' to encourage those who continue to smoke to consider quitting.

The primary care health team has a major role in the diagnosis and management of COPD, usually being responsible for the care of all but the most severe cases. It is therefore important that primary healthcare teams comprise members trained in the prevention, recognition and treatment of the disease. Appropriately trained team members can facilitate management of COPD in the community, which is effective, integrated across all members of the providing team, in keeping with current guidelines and acceptable to the patient.

## Quality Outcomes Framework

The Quality Outcomes Framework (QOF) of the UK GP contract continues to recognise the importance of good management of COPD in primary care; this defines a set of clinical indicators based on current best available evidence. These indices look at the diagnosis and monitoring of disease, together with provision of strategies to prevent progression and acute exacerbations. The current QOF defines clinical indicators in the areas of identification of patients with COPD, recording of data relating to these patients and patient management, all of which are underpinned by current guidelines. Most GPs and primary healthcare teams already have systems in place which address these areas and the QOF is a means of ensuring they are constantly updated and all information is both current and accurate.

## Identification of patients

The diagnosis of COPD is most likely to occur in the community; consider it in all patients over the age of 35 who have a history of smoking. The primary care health team is well placed to identify patients with COPD during screening or new patient visits and during any interactions where a smoking history is routinely taken. The use of a health questionnaire can aid with the screening process. The team might also be able to identify a pattern of symptoms from clinical contacts, such as recurrent cough or episodes of breathlessness or wheeze. This can be particularly useful as symptoms taken in isolation are only of limited usefulness in making or excluding a diagnosis of COPD, while there is currently no single diagnostic test available. Where the history raises the suspicion that a patient may have COPD, perform a clinical examination and arrange spirometry. Ways to confidently make the diagnosis of COPD are described in detail in Chapter 4. Diagnosing or even raising the possibility of a diagnosis of COPD allows for a useful discussion with patients about smoking cessation in a way that is immediately relevant to them. Providing advice and support for smoking cessation at this time may help the patient to make a

*ABC of COPD*, Third Edition. Edited by Graeme P. Currie.
© 2017 John Wiley & Sons Ltd. Published 2017 by John Wiley & Sons Ltd.

decision to attempt to quit. Early diagnosis allows for the most effective management and potentially greater health benefits, particularly if the patient is able to stop smoking.

## Spirometry

In patients in whom a diagnosis of COPD is suspected, spirometry is vital to confirm airflow obstruction; the QOF for Primary Care indicates that this should be performed after the patient has received inhaled bronchodilators. National and international guidelines recommend its use in community settings both for the diagnosis and in guiding management of COPD. The availability of low-cost, portable, user-friendly machines means that spirometry can now be used as the standard measurement of lung function in the majority of primary care settings and replaces less useful and less informative peak expiratory flow measurements.

Spirometry must be performed by staff trained in the maintenance of equipment and how to correctly produce accurate and reproducible measurements. Individuals in the community who perform spirometry should receive initial (and regular) training and updates (Figure 14.1). In patients with clinical and spirometry evidence typical of COPD, bronchodilator reversibility testing is not required.

## Follow-up of stable COPD in the community

Many patients with COPD require regular contact with community medical services; those with stable disease may not seek help, but offer them a routine review appointment to assess their disease and treatment. Current guidelines suggest that those with mild-to-moderate disease should be reviewed and their disease assessed at least annually, while planned review of those with more severe COPD should take place at least twice a year and possibly more frequently as need dictates. Arrange

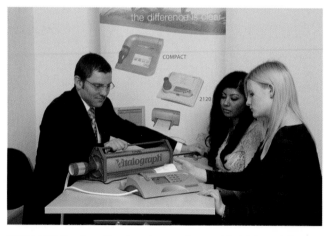

**Figure 14.1** Good-quality spirometry recordings and their interpretation can only be obtained by regular training and updates, delivered by suitably trained professional staff.

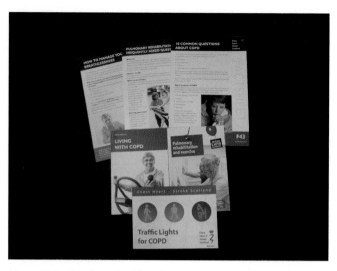

**Figure 14.2** All patients should receive written education about COPD and the management strategies involved.

review 4–6 weeks after a change in treatment or within a few weeks of an exacerbation. The following topics should usually be covered:

- smoking status
- symptom control
- treatment regime and concordance
- signs/symptoms of complications
- any additional input required
- examination
- spirometry
- assessment of breathlessness (using Modified Medical Research Council (MMRC) scale)
- pulse oximetry (if available)
- nutritional state (body mass index (BMI) calculation)
- mental state: is there evidence of anxiety or depression?
- vaccination status
- patient education (such as knowledge of the disease, treatments and inhaler technique) (Figure 14.2).

Reviews should take place with those team members who specialise in the treatment of COPD; this may include GPs, practice nurses, health visitors, community physiotherapists, community pharmacists, occupational therapists and nurse specialists. Because of the number of team members who may be involved in the care of an individual, it is important that all members have knowledge of the management plan in use and are able to share information with each other. Using a single set of electronic records which can be accessed by all relevant healthcare professionals will most easily facilitate this.

## Organisation of care at a practice level

The General Medical Services contract for GPs in the UK includes a set of QOF indicators for COPD. These are reviewed on a regular basis and are underpinned by current guidelines.

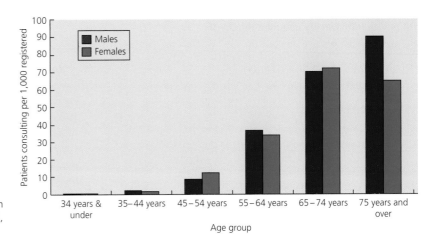

**Figure 14.3** Estimated number of patients in Scotland consulting a GP or practice nurse for COPD at least once in the financial year 2012–2013 per 1000 patients registered, by gender and age. Source: ISD Scotland.

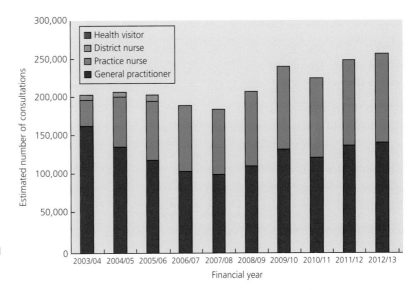

**Figure 14.4** Estimated number of consultations with a GP or practice-employed nurse for COPD in Scotland in the financial years 2003–2004 to 2012–2013, by staff discipline. Source: ISD Scotland.

The level at which these indicators are achieved dictates the level of remuneration GPs receive for caring for patients with COPD. In order to achieve targets, many practices have revised their organisation of care in order that accurate, easily accessible records are kept and treatment is optimised for all patients. The QOF does not set out standards for best practice and care, but suggests a minimum standard that should be achievable by all well-organised practices.

In order to meet the QOF indicators for COPD, a practice must be able to produce a register of all patients who have been diagnosed with the condition. The majority of patients should have had their diagnosis confirmed by postbronchodilator spirometry in a period from 3 months before the diagnosis was made up to 12 months afterwards. In order to meet the minimum standard, the majority of patients should have their forced expiratory volume in 1 second ($FEV_1$) and oxygen saturation recorded in any 12-month period together with an assessment of their degree of breathlessness using the MMRC dyspnoea score (see Chapter 3). Check inhaler technique (and correct where

necessary) at least annually. The majority of patients must also have been vaccinated against influenza each year; although not specifically outlined in the 2015–2016 QOF indicators for COPD, guidelines do recommend that pneumococcal vaccination should also be offered. The majority of GPs have easily achieved these standards for some time, although the need to demonstrate that they are actually met has led to many practices revisiting the way in which care is delivered and recorded (Figures 14.3, 14.4).

## National strategy

The first outcomes strategy for COPD in England was published in 2011. Its purpose was to set out ways by which healthcare outcomes to equal the best in the world might be achieved for COPD in England. A companion document published in 2012 recognised the importance of providing effective co-ordinated care by trained members of healthcare teams and draws on the quality standards for COPD as defined by NICE (Box 14.1).

1 People with COPD have one or more indicative symptoms recorded, and have the diagnosis confirmed by postbronchodilator spirometry carried out on calibrated equipment by healthcare professionals competent in its performance and interpretation

2 People with COPD have a current individualised comprehensive management plan, which includes high-quality information and educational material about the condition and its management, relevant to the stage of disease

3 People with COPD are offered inhaled and oral therapies, in accordance with NICE guidance, as part of an individualised comprehensive management plan

4 People with COPD have a comprehensive clinical and psychosocial assessment, at least once a year or more frequently if indicated, which includes degree of breathlessness, frequency of exacerbations, validated measures of health status and prognosis, presence of hypoxia and co-morbidities

5 People with COPD who smoke are regularly encouraged to stop and are offered the full range of evidence-based smoking cessation support

6 People with COPD meeting appropriate criteria are offered an effective, timely and accessible multidisciplinary pulmonary rehabilitation programme

7 People who have had an exacerbation of COPD are provided with individualised written advice on early recognition of future exacerbations, management strategies (including appropriate provision of antibiotics and corticosteroids for self-treatment at home) and a named contact

8 People with COPD potentially requiring long-term oxygen therapy are assessed in accordance with NICE guidance by a specialist oxygen service

9 People with COPD receiving long-term oxygen therapy are reviewed in accordance with NICE guidance, at least annually, by a specialist oxygen service

10 People admitted to hospital with an exacerbation of COPD are cared for by a respiratory team, and have access to a specialist early supported-discharge scheme with appropriate community support

11 People admitted to hospital with an exacerbation of COPD and with persistent acidotic ventilator failure are promptly assessed for, and receive, non-invasive ventilation delivered by appropriately trained staff in a dedicated setting

12 People admitted to hospital with an exacerbation of COPD are reviewed within 2 weeks of discharge

13 People with advanced COPD, and their carers, are identified and offered palliative care that addresses physical, social and emotional needs

## Smoking cessation

Health professionals in the community are ideally placed to assist patients in smoking cessation; successfully encouraging a patient with COPD to stop smoking is one of the most valuable interventions that can be made in a primary care setting. Smoking cessation is the single most effective and cost-effective intervention to both reduce the risk of developing COPD and stop its further progression. Primary care practitioners should not only concentrate their

efforts on patients who have already developed COPD, but should also seek to help all patients who smoke irrespective of their age and should keep a record of their efforts and outcomes.

Routinely take a smoking history in all new patients and in any patient with symptoms of a possible smoking-related disease. The current UK QOF recognises the part that smoking plays in ill health and rewards practices for recording smoking status in the past 12 months in individuals with a number of chronic diseases (including COPD). It also rewards efforts in supporting patients who smoke to quit using a strategy that includes (as a minimum) the provision of literature and appropriate therapy (see Chapter 5). The QOF indicates that patients over the age of 15 years recorded as current smokers should be offered support and treatment at least once every 2 years to encourage them to stop and that a record of these efforts should be kept. For those who have smoking-related conditions, the QOF asks for a record to be kept of patients who have had an offer of support to stop smoking in the preceding 12 months.

Most patients are fully aware of the adverse effects of smoking in general terms, and 'lectures' on problems that may occur in the future are unlikely to be effective in producing change. Instead, assess patients' readiness to change their behaviour; a framework to use as an assessment tool is the States of Change model (Figure 14.5). This describes the four stages involved in making a change in behaviour together with maintenance or relapse. Knowing which stage a patient has reached allows more appropriate discussions to take place and an open question such as 'Have you ever tried to give up?' allows you to determine where on the model a patient is at any particular time.

In 2012, the National Centre for Smoking Cessation and Training published guidelines on best practice for training those involved in assisting patients to stop smoking. These suggest that help to patients should include offers of behavioural counselling, group therapy, pharmacotherapy or a combination of treatments that have been

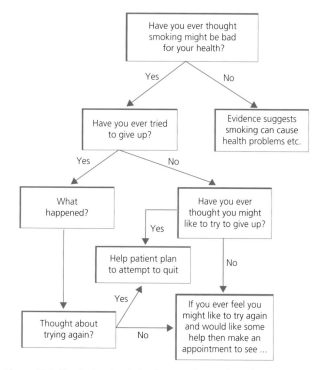

**Figure 14.5** Simple structured plan for assessing readiness for an attempt to stop smoking.

shown to be effective. The guidelines state that support, counselling and advice about smoking cessation should be tailored to the needs of individuals, particularly those from minority, ethnic and disadvantaged groups, and should be provided in a language chosen by patients wherever possible. Ideally, each practice would have at least one member of staff who has received training in line with these guidelines and whose knowledge in the area is maintained. Where this is not possible, refer patients to a local or regional centre in order to receive assistance and support in line with current best practice.

## Referral for specialist opinion

The decision to refer for a specialist opinion may occur at any stage in the disease. This will also depend on the individual primary care provider's experience, available facilities and confidence in managing COPD. Reasons for specialist referral include:
- diagnostic uncertainty
- patient choice
- assessment of suitability for domiciliary oxygen therapy, provision of a nebuliser or domiciliary non-invasive ventilation
- severe airflow obstruction
- marked functional impairment
- rapidly declining lung function
- assessment of suitability of domiciliary oxygen in hypoxic patients
- young age or family history of α1-antitrypsin deficiency
- persistent symptoms despite apparent adequate therapy
- frequent exacerbations and infections
- haemoptysis or suspected lung cancer
- presence of signs suggestive of cor pulmonale
- assessment and consideration of oral corticosteroids, lung volume reduction surgery, lung transplantation, bullectomy
- referral to a specialist stop smoking practitioner
- assessment for pulmonary rehabilitation where no process allowing direct referral exists.

## Management of stable disease

This is discussed in Chapters 6, 7 and 8.

## Management of acute exacerbations

The definition and clinical features of an acute exacerbation are described in Chapter 12. Most patients with an acute exacerbation of COPD do not require hospital admission and can be successfully managed in the community (Table 14.1). The number of exacerbations a patient experiences is likely to increase as the severity of the disease increases; patients and those living with them should have access to a clear and detailed written plan describing how to respond to worsening respiratory symptoms. Such a plan should contain information on:
- how to recognise an exacerbation
- what treatment to take and its anticipated duration (antibiotics, oral corticosteroids and increase in bronchodilators)
- who to contact in an emergency with contact details (including out-of-hours services or the nearest emergency department)
- how to recognise when emergency services should be contacted.
    In addition to a written plan, it is often appropriate to provide patients with a 'just in case' box, especially for individuals who

**Table 14.1** Factors to consider when deciding where to most suitably manage a patient with an acute exacerbation of COPD.

| Factor | Favours home care | Favours admission |
|---|---|---|
| Able to look after themselves | Yes | No |
| Degree of breathlessness | Mild | Severe |
| General condition | Good | Worsening |
| Level of consciousness | Normal | Confused or impaired conscious level |
| Rate of onset | Gradual | Rapid |
| Using long-term oxygen therapy | No | Yes |
| Social circumstances | Good | Less than ideal |
| Significant co-morbidity, e.g. heart disease, insulin-dependent diabetes | No | Yes |
| Oxygen saturation | >90% | <90% |
| Cyanosis | No | Yes |
| Worsening oedema | No | Yes |
| Community team available to support care at home if required | Yes | No |

experience frequent exacerbations. This contains drugs for use in an exacerbation, with instructions to alert their primary care team at the earliest opportunity whenever they have had recourse to use it. It facilitates quick access to treatment and allows the primary care team to make arrangements to check on the patient's health each time the box is used.

Investigations are not usually required during an acute exacerbation of COPD in the community, and sputum culture is not routinely recommended. Pulse oximetry may be a useful indicator of the severity of an episode and in some cases the patient and/or their carers can be supplied with an oximeter, providing appropriate education and training have been given.

Management of an acute exacerbation most usually involves 7–14 days of prednisolone 30–40 mg/day, broad-spectrum antibiotics (especially if sputum is more purulent and of greater quantity than usual in association with increased breathlessness), regular use of inhaled bronchodilators and with continuation of all other inhaled and oral treatments. Some patients may also find short-term use of a nebuliser to deliver bronchodilators of benefit, especially when too breathless to use hand-held devices. Patients living alone or with difficult social circumstances may require admission to a community facility (where this is an option) or an enhanced domiciliary care package may be put in place. Many exacerbations can also be easily managed in the community following brief assessment at hospital by way of immediate, early or assisted discharge schemes. Following an exacerbation, the recovery of the patient should be monitored in order to detect failure to improve and ensure measures are considered to try and prevent further exacerbations. When it is agreed by all health professionals that the final stages of COPD have been reached and that a patient is no longer responsive to medical therapy, palliative care may be offered in either the community or hospice setting (see Chapter 15). Palliative care and support should be provided for these patients and carers by the full range of community healthcare team members similar to any other terminal disease.

## Further reading

Decramer M, Janssens W, Miravitlles M. chronic obstructive pulmonary disease. *Lancet* 2012; **379**: 1341–1351.

Global Initiative for Chronic Obstructive Lung Disease (GOLD). Global Strategy for the Diagnosis, Management and Prevention of COPD. Available at: http://goldcopd.org/gold-2017-global-strategy-diagnosis-management-prevention-copd/ (accessed 24 February 2017).

National Centre for Smoking Cessation and Training. NCSCT Training Standard. Learning Outcomes for Training Stop Smoking Practitioners. Available at: www.ncsct.co.uk/usr/pub/NCSCT%20Training%20Standard. pdf (accessed 24 February 2017).

National Institute for Health and Care Excellence. CG101. Chronic obstructive pulmonary disease in over 16s: diagnosis and management. Available at: www.nice.org.uk/guidance/CG101 (accessed 26 February 2017).

National Institute for Health and Care Excellence. Chronic obstructive pulmonary disease in adults. QS10. Available at: www.nice.org.uk/guidance/qs10 (accessed 24 February 2017).

NHS Employers. 2015/16 General Medical Services (GMS) contract. Guidance for GMS contract 2015/16. Available at: http://www.nhsemployers.org/~/media/Employers/Documents/Primary%20care%20contracts/GMS/GMS%20guidance%202010-present/2015-16/201516%20GMS%20Guidance. pdf (accessed 24 February 2017)

www.MyLungsMyLife.org

# CHAPTER 15

# Death, Dying and End-of-Life Issues

*Gordon Linklater*

Highland Hospice, Inverness, UK

---

## OVERVIEW

- Chronic obstructive pulmonary disease (COPD) is a life-limiting disease.
- Distressing symptoms – such as breathlessness, fatigue, depression, anxiety and pain – are common in end-stage disease.
- End-of-life needs (such as uncontrolled symptoms, isolation and emotional distress) are often unmet.
- Effective symptom management requires a multidisciplinary and holistic approach.
- Non-drug strategies play a major role in dealing with most end-of-life symptoms.
- Morphine can help relieve persistent breathlessness; when carefully titrated against symptoms, it does not hasten death.
- Oxygen plays little or no role in relieving breathlessness in patients who do not fulfil criteria for long term oxygen therapy.
- Planning for end-of-life care should take place in parallel with life-prolonging treatments.
- Service development and improving access to palliative care are important areas to explore in both primary and secondary care.

---

Palliative care is defined as:

> *an approach that improves the quality of life of patients and their families, facing the problems associated with life-threatening illness, through the prevention and relief of suffering by means of early identification, assessment and treatment of pain and other problems: physical, psychosocial and spiritual.*

This approach requires care to be tailored to the individual needs of patients using the complementary skills of the multidisciplinary team.

Palliative care should ideally be accessible in all primary and secondary environments, irrespective of whether a diagnosis of cancer has been made. It is increasingly recognised that unmet needs prevent patients with end-stage chronic obstructive pulmonary disease (COPD) experiencing a 'good death'. Many barriers exist; examples include uncertain disease trajectory, lack of advance planning and knowledge of patient wishes, along with infrastructure and resource limitations. Nevertheless, healthcare providers and all other stakeholders should explore these issues in an attempt to improve the quality of care that is available for such patients.

COPD is the most common respiratory disorder which requires palliation of symptoms. Its disease trajectory – usually punctuated by exacerbations resulting in peaks and troughs in levels of functioning, symptoms, quality of life and well-being – differs from that of lung cancer and dementia/general frailty (Figure 15.1).

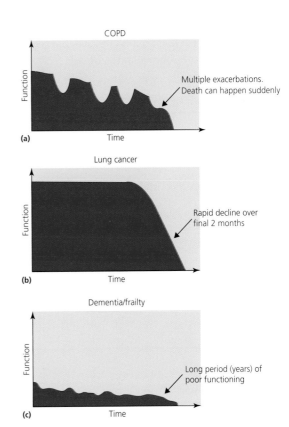

**Figure 15.1** Typical disease trajectories in patients with COPD, lung cancer and dementia/general frailty.

---

*ABC of COPD*, Third Edition. Edited by Graeme P. Currie.
© 2017 John Wiley & Sons Ltd. Published 2017 by John Wiley & Sons Ltd.

## When do patients enter a palliative phase?

Accurately predicting the prognosis of COPD is impossible. Indeed, exacerbations are a common occurrence and it is difficult to judge which one will ultimately result in death. These episodic deteriorations can be life threatening, but may also respond quickly and dramatically to intensive treatment, with patients returning to previous levels of health and function, even in those with advanced disease. However, when it does occur during an exacerbation, death can seem sudden and unexpected to some families.

The presence or absence of some clinical features may help guide discussions to some extent (Table 15.1). Unlike many cancers, there is no clear cut-off threshold to indicate when disease-modifying treatments are no longer appropriate. Instead, a model of care is needed where poor long-term prognosis is acknowledged and symptoms are controlled even while treatments aimed at prolonging life are implemented, with a focus on preserving individual quality of life.

## Maintaining quality of life

Quality of life is difficult to define on an individual basis. In general, health-related quality of life deteriorates as a chronic disease progresses. For many patients, particularly those who are aware that they have a life-limiting illness, factors that influence individual quality of life tend not to be biomedical, but reflect issues of control and interpersonal relationships (Table 15.2). Most patients, therefore, find open and honest discussion about end-of-life issues and involvement in decision making to be worthwhile and beneficial.

**Table 15.1** Predictors of poor prognosis.

| General (≥2 of) | Factors related to COPD (≥1 of) |
|---|---|
| • Poor or declining performance status with limited reversibility<br>• Dependent on others for most care needs due to physical health problems<br>• ≥2 unplanned hospital admissions in previous 6 months<br>• Weight loss (5–10% over 3–6 months)<br>• Persistent troublesome symptoms despite optimum treatment of underlying illness<br>• Patient requests palliative/ supportive care or treatment withdrawal | • Breathless at rest or minimal exertion between exacerbations<br>• Previous non-invasive ventilation for hypercapnic respiratory failure or intubation and mechanical ventilation contraindicated<br>• Fulfils long-term oxygen therapy criteria |

**Table 15.2** Some of the factors which influence quality of life.

| Enhanced by | Diminished by |
|---|---|
| Maintaining control | Losing independence |
| Family member access | Feeling a burden |
| Hobbies/activity involvement | Lost activities, hobbies, employment |
| Caring attitude of staff | Pain or fear of pain |
| Feeling safe/not alone | |
| Pleasing and comfortable physical environment | |

## Symptom control

The most commonly reported distressing symptoms in advanced COPD are:

• breathlessness
• fatigue
• anxiety
• pain
• depression
• insomnia
• anorexia
• constipation.

The best symptom control is achieved if it is both possible and appropriate to treat the underlying cause of the symptom. However, in life-limiting illness this cannot always be achieved. Non-drug approaches are useful, underused and should preferentially be explored prior to the use of drugs.

## Breathlessness

The neurophysiology of breathlessness is complex and involves both the control of breathing through brainstem feedback loops and perception of breathlessness through higher cortical and limbic processing (Figure 15.2). Patients almost universally find breathlessness distressing, irrespective of its apparent severity. It is important to note that, strictly speaking, breathlessness is a symptom reported by the patient (and not a sign observed by the healthcare worker or family member).

### Treat underlying cause, if possible and appropriate

In COPD, particularly during exacerbations, antibiotics, steroids, bronchodilators and non-invasive ventilation (NIV) may all prove useful in relieving breathlessness, even when patients are very close to the end of life. Although NIV is generally regarded as a life-saving intervention, it can also be effectively used for palliation. For example,

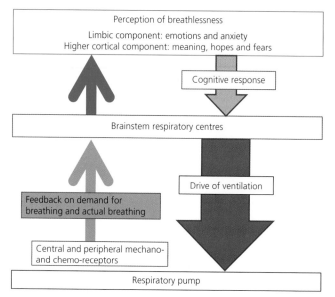

**Figure 15.2** Limbic and higher cognitive factors interact to influence the perception of breathlessness.

it can be useful in alleviating breathlessness and symptoms related to hypercapnia such as headache. It may also 'buy' the patient and relatives time, so that outstanding personal, family, financial and psychosocial matters can be openly discussed. However, avoid prolonged and futile use of NIV, especially when any respiratory acidosis fails to resolve after prolonged treatment. Consider and treat other causes of breathlessness such as anaemia, pulmonary oedema, pulmonary emboli, intercurrent infection, anxiety and atrial fibrillation.

## Non-drug approaches

Encourage an upright posture with shoulders supported to promote abdominal breathing and recruitment of accessory muscles (see Chapter 6, Figure 6.4). Other non-drug strategies such as reassurance, distraction (e.g. family visits, television, art classes), adapting daily activities, energy conservation and relaxation classes are helpful and inexpensive (Figure 15.3). The sensation of air blowing across the face can reduce the perception of breathlessness, while some patients benefit from being positioned beside an open window (Figure 15.4). A hand-held fan can be a cheap and effective way of giving a patient some control; advise them to have the stream of air blowing from the side rather than directly into the face.

There is little or no evidence supporting the use of 'short-burst' (or regular) oxygen in relatively non-hypoxic patients with breathlessness. Moreover, oxygen can lead to psychological dependence and 'medicalisation' of a preterminal event. Other potential harms include limiting movement and restricting activities due to the cumbersome nature of oxygen delivery devices and tubing, anxiety/worry occurring during short-term disruption of supply, social stigma, drying of the nasal mucosa and cost.

Many individuals describe particular difficulty with 'getting a breath in', especially in the context of anxiety and panic. Encourage patients to concentrate on breathing control, specifically asking them to breathe out fully (Figure 15.5), which can help reduce hyperinflation and make inhalation easier. Physiotherapists are useful in instructing patients in such techniques.

Breathlessness almost inevitably reduces functional ability and can lead to a sense of loss of control. Energy conservation

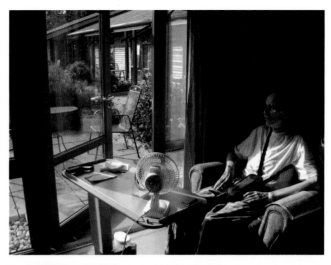

**Figure 15.4** An open window or bedside fan can help reduce the sensation of breathlessness; a fan blowing air across the face may be of even greater benefit.

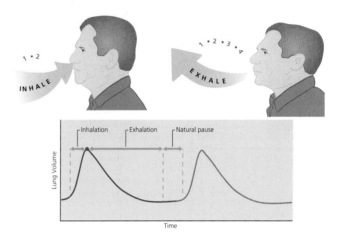

**Figure 15.5** Focusing on longer 'outbreaths' can reduce breathlessness and panic.

techniques, functional aids (e.g. walking aids, bed levers, raised seats) and appropriate social care can all allow patients to maintain functional independence to some degree.

## Palliative drug approaches

For patients with end-stage disease who experience persistent breathlessness despite maximal treatment and non-drug strategies, have a low threshold for starting opioids (Box 15.1). Careful titration of opioids will not hasten death. Less evidence exists for benzodiazepines in the management of breathlessness (Box 15.2), but in clinical practice they are often helpful when managing patients who experience significant anxiety associated with breathlessness (Figure 15.6).

Box 15.1 **Use of opioids in end-stage COPD.**

- Reduce the sensation of breathlessness
- Initially use oral morphine (e.g. morphine 2.5–5 mg every 4 hours as required, with carefully titrated doses)
- Modified-release morphine preparations can be useful to control 'background' breathlessness

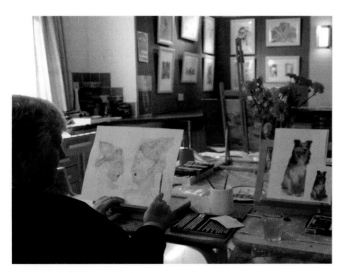

**Figure 15.3** Distractions, pleasurable and stimulating activities and a calm, relaxing environment can improve quality of life in those with advanced COPD.

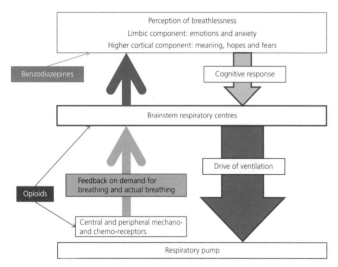

**Figure 15.6** Opioids and benzodiazepines can influence the limbic and higher cognitive factors that contribute to the perception of breathlessness.

## Fatigue

Fatigue is highly prevalent in all life-limiting illnesses. Try to identify underlying causes and treat whenever possible (for example, anaemia, hypothyroidism, poor sleep hygiene, depression, excessive alcohol intake and excessive sedative drugs). Non-drug approaches provide the mainstay of treatment. Measures to improve sleep quality and length include reserving the bedroom for sleeping only (e.g. removing a television), avoiding caffeine-containing drinks in the evening and use of blackout curtains, etc. Occupational therapist and physiotherapist interventions can be useful; examples include graded exercise programmes, use of energy conservation techniques and provision of aids for activities of daily living. Palliative drug treatments for fatigue are usually ineffective.

## Depression and anxiety

Depression is underdiagnosed and undertreated in patients with advanced COPD. Untreated depression makes dealing with other physical or psychosocial issues more difficult. While many symptoms of depression are present in advanced physical disease (fatigue, loss of appetite and disturbed sleep), feelings of worthlessness or inappropriate guilt are highly suggestive of an

underlying depressive disorder. A good screening test is simply to ask 'Are you depressed?'. Several classes of antidepressants are available.

- Sertraline (initial dose 50 mg at night, titrated by 50 mg every 2 weeks to a maximum dose of 200 mg once daily) – may cause gastrointestinal upset.
- Amitriptyline (initial dose 10–25 mg at night, titrated cautiously to 75–150 mg at night) – useful if sedation is required or neuropathic pain is a problem; anticholinergic side effects commonly limit dose titration, particularly in the elderly.
- Mirtazapine (initial dose 15 mg at night, titrated by 15 mg a week to 45 mg at night) – useful if patient is anxious; may also help neuropathic pain and stimulate appetite.

Anxiety is common near the end of life, and is exacerbated by feeling out of control or other significant symptoms, particularly breathlessness. Benzodiazepines are the mainstays of drug treatment, although sedative antidepressants can also be useful.

## Pain

Chest pain is often found in advanced and end-stage COPD, although it tends to be often overlooked and undertreated. It can be caused by respiratory muscle fatigue, rib fractures due to coughing, osteoporosis and pleural infection. Regular paracetamol and non-steroidal anti-inflammatory drugs with the addition of regular oral morphine for moderate to severe pain are the mainstays of treatment. The use of heat pads, cold pads and transcutaneous electrical nerve stimulation (TENS) machines can be helpful. Different pain types may also respond to different treatment modalities; for example, for neuropathic pain consider tricyclic antidepressants or anticonvulsants, and for an osteoporotic rib fracture, consider an intercostal nerve block (Figures 15.7, 15.8).

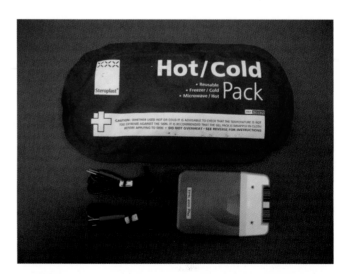

**Figure 15.7** Hot/cold pads and TENS machines are useful adjuvants for pain control.

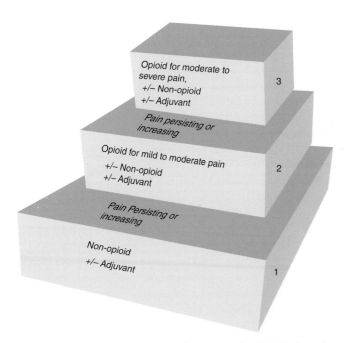

**Figure 15.8** World Health Organization three-step analgesic ladder. Examples of non-opioids include paracetamol and non-steroidal anti-inflammatory drugs, weak opioids include codeine and tramadol, strong opioids include morphine, oxycodone and fentanyl. Adjuvants include other drugs to help with pain management such as those used for neuropathic pain and those used to counteract adverse effects.

## Advance care planning

Similar proportions of patients with COPD and lung cancer opt for 'comfort care' versus 'life-prolonging care', although those with COPD are less likely to have end-of-life discussions with healthcare professionals. Most patients with COPD harbour fears about the progression of their disease and desire more information. Discussion about the dying process allows patients to choose what arrangements should be made to manage the final stages of their illness, and to attend to personal and other concerns considered important towards the end of life. Ideally, this should take place prior to the terminal event. Try to engage patients and their carers to discuss (and record) what treatments they would (and would not) like in the event of a deterioration; these may include transfer to hospital and management options such as antibiotics, corticosteroids, non-invasive ventilation, arterial blood gases, arterial lines and transfer to high-dependency and intensive care units.

Decisions about withholding or withdrawing life-prolonging treatment can be difficult and distressing. However, it is important to be aware of the following.

- Competent adults may decide to refuse treatment even where refusal may result in harm to themselves or in their own death; clinicians are bound to respect a competent refusal of treatment.
- Where an adult patient has become incompetent, a refusal of treatment made when the patient was competent must be respected, provided it is clearly applicable to the present circumstances and there is no reason to believe that the patient had changed his/her mind.
- There is no obligation to give treatment that is futile and burdensome; in the context of end-stage COPD, cardiopulmonary resuscitation (CPR) has a negligible success rate.

- Final responsibility rests with the clinician to decide what treatments are clinically indicated; these should be provided subject to a competent patient's consent or, in the case of an incompetent patient, any known views of that patient prior to becoming incapacitated and taking account of the views offered by the family.
- Family members/carers/'next of kin' do not have decision-making rights or responsibilities for treatment consent/refusal (unless the patient has designated a proxy decision maker, e.g. a power of attorney).

## Advance refusal of treatment

Advance refusals of treatment – also known as 'living wills' or 'advance directives' – are legal documents that allow patients to indicate their preferences for care, should they no longer be able to make decisions due to illness or incapacity. An advance refusal of treatment can specify that under certain circumstances, the patient can withdraw consent for life-supporting interventions. Such a refusal is binding, as long as it clearly relates to the current circumstances. A patient can make an advance statement of preferences for treatment and care, but this statement cannot demand treatment that is deemed clinically inappropriate. An advance refusal may be invalid if:

- it does not relate to current circumstances
- there is reason to doubt authenticity
- it is felt that it was created under duress
- there is doubt as to the person's state of mind (at the time of signing).

If a patient is considering an advance refusal of treatment, encourage them to discuss its contents with family/carers and ensure that a copy is placed in their medical records. Legal advice, to help draft the form and provide a witness signature, may also be useful.

## Do not attempt cardiopulmonary resuscitation decisions

If cardiac or respiratory arrest is an expected part of the dying process and CPR will not be successful, an advance decision not to attempt CPR should be made and recorded. It is expected that the patient should be informed of this decision unless it is felt that they would come to serious harm as a result of receiving that information. Record these discussions in the patient's notes. If a patient decides that CPR would not be in their best interests, even if their clinician feels it may be successful, then an advance decision not to attempt CPR should also be recorded.

Advance decisions not to attempt CPR are typically recorded on a 'Do Not Attempt Cardiopulmonary Resuscitation' document. The form should be completed by the most senior clinician available (who may be a suitably qualified non-medical practitioner such as a specialist nurse). The document should not be filled in by a Foundation Year 1 (pre-registration) doctor. It should be kept where it will be easily accessed in the event of a sudden deterioration. It is important to remember that the form only relates to CPR. Decisions about other potential medical treatments (e.g. parenteral fluids, antibiotics and NIV) will need to be made and recorded separately, for example on a treatment escalation plan or 'ceiling of care' document in the case notes. When a patient moves between care environments, these documents should travel with them. The ongoing appropriateness of the Do Not Attempt CPR decision should be reviewed as soon as practical in the new environment.

## Ways to engage patients in end-of-life discussions

There is little doubt that knowing when, where and how to engage patients in discussions about end of life care is challenging. Patients often value having more information and being involved in decision making, although health professionals may avoid such discussions to avoid making themselves feel ill at ease and because of (possibly unfounded) fears of upsetting patients.

Consider end-of-life discussions when it is clinically apparent that the patient is at increased risk of death. For example, if the answer to the question 'Would I be surprised if this patient died in the next 6 months?' is no, then it is clear that planning for the possibility of end-of-life care is needed. A useful opportunity to initiate such a conversation with a patient is when they have just recovered from an exacerbation. They may have questions about what has just happened and are likely have strong views about what should happen if and when a future exacerbation occurs. It is much more difficult to have these conversations in the context of an acute exacerbation.

Health professionals who have these discussions should have sufficient clinical experience to discuss prognosis and treatment options. They should also have 'authority' to make clinical decisions and possess knowledge of the patient, their family and social context. This therefore needs good communication between primary and secondary care For example, if a general practitioner has end-of-life discussions, they require information regarding likely prognosis, treatment options and appropriate ceilings of care, while if the respiratory specialist has such a conversation, they would benefit from information relating to the patient's social circumstances and care available in the community.

Discussions should happen at the patient's pace and may need to be continued over several consultations. Good communication skills are necessary. Open questions such as: 'What would you like to ask me?' are generally more useful than closed questions such as: 'Do you have any questions?' (Box 15.3).

---

Box 15.3 **Potentially useful questions for end-of-life discussions.**

- 'How are you coping with your illness?'
- 'What are you thinking about the future?'
- 'What would you like to ask me about how things might go from here?'
- 'What things affect your quality of life?'
- 'Patients like you often find admissions to hospital frightening. How was that last admission for you?'
- If things become worse again:
  ○ 'Where would you like to be cared for?'
  ○ 'If that is not possible, what other options have you considered?'
  ○ 'What treatments do you want/not want?'
- 'What are you most worried about?'

---

## End-of-life care

Where the rapid progression of a patient's end-stage condition is likely, and death is considered an inevitable outcome, ensure that terminal care needs are identified and met appropriately. This should include consideration of wishes regarding the appropriate place for receiving care, which may affect treatment options available (e.g. home, care home, community hospital or general hospital), and the need for religious, spiritual, family or other personal support.

If patients are admitted to hospital, avoid unnecessary interventions (e.g. regular venepuncture, arterial blood gases, routine monitoring of vital signs). Discontinue inappropriate drugs (e.g. statins, antiplatelet drugs, bisphosphonates, heparin, proton pump inhibitors, etc.).

The most common symptoms in the terminal phase include pain, breathlessness, anxiety/agitation and copious respiratory secretions ('death rattle'). In anticipating these symptoms, prescribe 'as-required' medications early to allow rapid symptom control (Box 15.4). If several 'as-required' doses are needed, consider a 24-hour subcutaneous infusion via syringe driver to maintain symptom control. If the patient is at home, arrangements will be needed to ensure staff are available to administer such treatments over a 24-hour period.

---

Box 15.4 **Drugs used in terminal care.**

- Morphine 2.5 mg subcutaneous as required for pain or breathlessness*
- Midazolam 2.5 mg subcutaneous as required for agitation or breathlessness#
- Hyoscine butylbromide 20 mg subcutaneous as required for respiratory secretions

Notes: * if opioid naive. If not opioid naive, the dose should be half the oral 'breakthrough' dose of immediate-release morphine.
# Higher doses may be needed if the patient is already taking benzodiazepines.
Typical starting doses of the above subcutaneous drugs in a syringe driver are morphine 10 mg, midazolam 10 mg, hyoscine butylbromide 60 mg.

---

## Further reading

Fallon M, Hanks G. ABC of Palliative Care, 2nd edn. Blackwell Publishing, Oxford, 2006.

Gardiner C, Gott M, Small N et al. Living with advanced chronic obstructive pulmonary disease: patients concerns regarding death and dying. *Palliative Medicine* 2009; **23**: 691–697.

Joshi M, Joshi A, Bartter T. Symptom burden in chronic obstructive pulmonary disease and cancer. *Current Opinion in Pulmonary Medicine* 2012; **18**: 97–103.

Solano J, Gomes B, Higginson I. A comparison of symptom prevalence in far advanced cancer, AIDS, heart disease, chronic obstructive pulmonary disease and renal disease. *Journal of Pain and Symptom Management* 2006; **31**: 58–69.

Spathis A, Booth S. End of life care in chronic obstructive pulmonary disease: in search of a good death. *International Journal of Chronic Obstructive Pulmonary Disease* 2008; **3**: 11–29.

www.palliativecareguidelines.scot.nhs.uk/

www.palliativedrugs.com/palliative-care-formulary.html

www.spict.org.uk/

www.gmc-uk.org/guidance/current/library/witholding_lifeprolonging_guidance.asp

www.gmc-uk.org/static/documents/content/Treatment_and_care_towards_the_end_of_life_-_English_1015.pdf

## CHAPTER 16

# Future Treatments

*Peter J. Barnes*

National Heart and Lung Institute, Imperial College London, London, UK

---

**OVERVIEW**

- Effective drug development in chronic obstructive pulmonary disease (COPD) is challenging because of a variety of methodological issues relating to clinical trials.
- Once-daily long-acting inhaled bronchodilators (alone or in combination) are now the mainstay of pharmacological treatment.
- More effective smoking cessation strategies are in varying degrees of development.
- Specially designed anti-inflammatory agents and mediator antagonists have been difficult to develop.

Current therapy for the treatment of chronic obstructive pulmonary disease (COPD) is often less than ideal and fails to reduce the relentless decline in lung function that leads to increasing symptoms, disability and exacerbations or impact upon mortality. Scientists and pharmaceutical companies continue their quest to seek more effective therapies that may control or even reverse the underlying disease process.

## The continuing challenge of drug development

Multiple reasons explain why drug development in COPD proves to be difficult. For example:

- the molecular and cell biology of COPD is still poorly understood, although there has been increasing research and important advances in this area, leading to the identification of new therapeutic targets
- animal models of COPD for early drug testing (usually smoking mice) are unsatisfactory as they fail to mimic all the features of the disease, particularly small airway fibrosis and exacerbations
- uncertainty exists about which biomarkers in blood, sputum or breath may predict clinical efficacy or disease progression
- methodological uncertainties exist about how best to evaluate drugs for COPD in the long term, although there is increasing

interest in patient-reported outcome measures, since changes in forced expiratory volume in 1 second ($FEV_1$) poorly reflect clinical improvements
- many patients with COPD have important co-morbidities – such as ischaemic heart disease, cardiac failure, hypertension and diabetes mellitus – which may exclude them from clinical trials of new therapies and therefore create uncertainty regarding the usefulness of some drugs in 'real life'.

However, despite all these issues, progress is under way and several new classes of drugs are now in preclinical and clinical stages of development.

## New bronchodilators

The mainstay of current drug therapy in COPD is long-acting bronchodilators. Long-acting muscarinic antagonists (LAMAs) and long-acting $\beta_2$-agonists (LABAs) are the preferred first-line agents in symptomatic individuals with established disease (Box 16.1). LABAs and LAMAs appear to confer additive bronchodilator effects, so that fixed combination inhalers containing both classes of drug are now available and others are in development. As well as being formulated with LAMAs, some of the newer LABAs have been formulated to be given with inhaled corticosteroids in the same inhaler device. Moreover, dual function molecules that exert both LAMA and LABA activity are being evaluated in clinical trials. Although there has been a search for novel classes of bronchodilators – such as potassium channel openers and 'bitter taste' receptor agonists – these have proved to be less effective than established bronchodilators and exhibit more adverse effects.

Box 16.1 **Current and future long-acting bronchodilators for the treatment of COPD.**

**Long-acting $\beta_2$-agonists**
- Salmeterol (twice daily)
- Formoterol (twice daily)
- Indacaterol (once daily)

---

*ABC of COPD*, Third Edition. Edited by Graeme P. Currie.
© 2017 John Wiley & Sons Ltd. Published 2017 by John Wiley & Sons Ltd.

- Vilanterol (once daily)*
- Olodaterol (once daily)

**Long-acting anticholinergics**
- Tiotropium bromide (once daily)
- Glycopyrronium bromide (once daily)
- Umeclidinium bromide (once daily)
- Aclidinium bromide (twice daily)

**Combination inhalers**
- Salmeterol/fluticasone propionate (Seretide: twice daily)
- Formoterol/budesonide (Symbicort or Duoresp Spiromax: twice daily)
- Formoterol/beclomethasone (Fostair: twice daily)
- Vilanterol/fluticasone furoate (Relvar: once daily)
- Indacaterol/mometasone furoate (QMF149: once daily)
- Indacaterol/glycopyrronium bromide (Ultibro: once daily)
- Vilanterol/umeclidinium bromide (Anoro: once daily)
- Olodaterol/tiotropium bromide (Spiolto: once daily)

**Muscarinic antagonist/β-agonist (MABA)**
- GSK-961081

* Can only be administered as a combination inhaler (with umeclidinium or fluticasone furoate).

Combination inhalers that contain an inhaled corticosteroid plus a LABA are commonly prescribed for patients with more advanced COPD. Both salmeterol plus fluticasone (Seretide) and formoterol plus budesonide (Symbicort) are more effective than their separate constituents as monotherapy, and are indicated in patients with more advanced airflow obstruction ($FEV_1 < 50\%$ predicted) who have frequent exacerbations ($\geq 2$ per year). A fixed combination inhaler containing a once-daily corticosteroid (fluticasone furoate) and long-acting $\beta_2$-agonist (vilanterol) is now also available.

## More effective smoking cessation strategies

Cigarette smoking is the major cause of COPD globally and quitting at most stages of the disease reduces disease progression. Smoking cessation is therefore an integral part of management, although current cessation strategies have had only limited long-term success. One of the most effective current aids to smoking cessation is the partial nicotine agonist varenicline, which targets the $\alpha_4\beta_2$ nicotinic acetylcholine receptor. Although varenicline is more effective than bupropion and nicotine replacement therapy, it still only achieves a quit rate of approximately 20% in 1 year and adverse effects – such as nausea and depression – may limit its use. Another approach which may have longer term benefits is the development of a vaccine against nicotine. This stimulates the production of antibodies that bind nicotine, meaning that it is unable to enter the brain. Several nicotine vaccines are currently undergoing evaluation in clinical trials, as are several other pharmacological approaches, but there is no evidence to date that they produce long-term smoking cessation (Box 16.2).

Box 16.2 **Current and future drugs for smoking cessation.**

**Current therapies**
- Nicotine replacement therapy
- Bupropion
- Varenicline ($\alpha_4\beta_2$ partial nicotine agonist)

**Future therapies**
- Nicotine vaccination (e.g. nic-Vax)
- Cannabinoid $CB_1$-receptor antagonists (e.g. rimonabant)
- $GABA_B$ antagonists
- Dopamine $D_3$ antagonists

## Treating pulmonary inflammation

Chronic obstructive pulmonary disease is characterised by chronic inflammation – particularly involving the small airways and lung parenchyma. The pattern of inflammation is different from that of asthma, with a predominance of macrophages, neutrophils and cytotoxic T-lymphocytes and different inflammatory mediators being involved. In contrast to asthma, the inflammation is largely resistant to the anti-inflammatory effects of corticosteroids, which has prompted the search for alternative anti-inflammatory therapies. Indeed, better understanding of the underlying mechanisms in COPD has led to the development of several potential therapeutic targets.

## Mediator antagonists

Many mediators, including lipid mediators and cytokines, are implicated in the pathophysiology of COPD. Inhibiting specific mediators, by receptor antagonists or synthesis inhibitors, is a relatively easy approach. However, doing so is unlikely to produce effective drugs, since so many mediators with similar effects are involved. Currently, several mediator antagonists are in clinical development. This is based on research demonstrating that the particular mediator level is increased in COPD, and in turn mimics some of the effects observed (Table 16.1). Antitumour necrosis factor antibodies are currently used to treat patients with severe rheumatoid arthritis and inflammatory bowel disease, but have been ineffective in COPD and may be associated with an increased risk of pneumonia and lung cancer. An interleukin-8 blocking antibody also appears to be largely ineffective. More promising strategies are small molecule antagonists of the chemokine receptor CXCR2, which mediates the effects of interleukin-8 and related chemokines. These drugs reduce neutrophilic inflammation in sputum in normal individuals after endotoxin and ozone challenge after oral administration, but have minimal clinical effects in long-term studies of COPD patients with a risk of neutropenia.

Oxidative stress is increased in COPD, particularly as the disease becomes more advanced and during exacerbations. Oxidative stress amplifies inflammation and may result in corticosteroid resistance and accelerated lung ageing, and is therefore a potentially important target for future therapies. Current antioxidants are not very effective, but more potent and stable antioxidants – such as analogues of superoxide dismutase and activators of the transcription factor Nrf2, which regulates several antioxidant genes – are now in development.

**Table 16.1** Mediator antagonists for potential use in COPD.

| Mediator | Major effect | Inhibitor |
|---|---|---|
| Leukotriene $B_4$ | Neutrophil chemotaxis | $BLT_1$-receptor antagonists (e.g. BIIL284) 5'-lipoxygenase inhibitors |
| Interleukin-8 | Neutrophil chemotaxis | Blocking antibodies (e.g. ABX-IL8) CXCR2 antagonists (e.g. Sch527123) |
| Interleukin-1β | Amplifying inflammation | Blocking antibodies (e.g. canakinumab) |
| Interleukin-6 | Amplifying inflammation | Blocking receptor antibody (e.g. tocilizumab) |
| Tumour necrosis factor-α | Amplifying inflammation | Blocking antibodies (e.g. infliximab) Soluble receptors (e.g. etanercept) |
| Epidermal growth factor | Mucus hypersecretion | EGFR kinase inhibitors (e.g. gefitinib) |
| Oxidative stress | Amplifying inflammation | Antioxidants (e.g. superoxide dismutase analogues) |
| | Steroid resistance | |
| Nitrative stress | Steroid resistance | Inducible NO synthase inhibitors (e.g. GSK-274150) |

## Protease inhibitors

Several proteases such as elastases – which are implicated in alveolar destruction – are a target for therapy in patients with COPD with marked emphysema. Proteases may be inhibited by giving endogenous antiproteases, such as α1-antitrypsin, or by small molecule protease inhibitors (Table 16.2). However, no clinical studies have yet demonstrated that these approaches have any beneficial effect.

**Table 16.2** Protease inhibitors for potential use in COPD.

| Protease inhibitor | Endogenous antiprotease | Small molecule |
|---|---|---|
| Neutrophil elastase | α1-Antitrypsin Secretory leukoprotease inhibitor Elafin | ONO-5046 |
| Cathepsins | Cystatins | Cysteine protease inhibitor |
| Matrix metalloproteinases MMP-9 | Tissue inhibitors of MMPs TIMP-1 | Marimastat MMP-9/12 selective (e.g. AZ11557272) |

## New anti-inflammatory treatments

Since corticosteroids are ineffective in reducing the inflammation found in COPD, alternative anti-inflammatory therapies are needed. The only new anti-inflammatory drug so far developed for COPD is the phosphodiesterase (PDE)-4 inhibitor roflumilast. PDE-4 inhibitors increase cyclic adenosine monophosphate concentrations in inflammatory cells and exhibit a broad spectrum of anti-inflammatory effects. Although effective in animal models of COPD, roflumilast has had limited success because of adverse effects, particularly nausea, diarrhoea and weight loss. However, roflumilast reduces exacerbations and improves lung function over 1 year, and provides benefit when added to long-acting bronchodilators and inhaled corticosteroids in COPD patients with $FEV_1 < 50\%$ predicted, chronic bronchitis and frequent exacerbations (Figures 16.1, 16.2). More selective inhibitors (PDE-4B inhibitors) and inhaled administration of these drugs are currently being investigated to circumvent the problem of adverse effects. Several other broad-spectrum anti-inflammatory therapies are currently under investigation (Box 16.3), although most of these are likely to be associated with adverse effects when given systemically, suggesting that inhaled administration may be required.

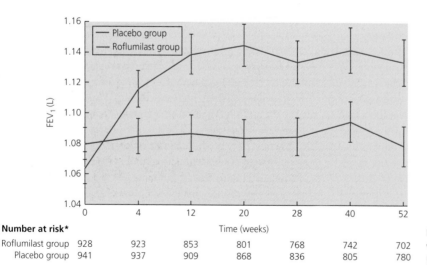

| Number at risk* | | | | | | | |
|---|---|---|---|---|---|---|---|
| Roflumilast group | 928 | 923 | 853 | 801 | 768 | 742 | 702 |
| Placebo group | 941 | 937 | 909 | 868 | 836 | 805 | 780 |

**Figure 16.1** Postbronchodilator $FEV_1$ in patients treated with roflumilast versus placebo over 52 weeks. Reproduced with permission from Martinez et al. (2015).

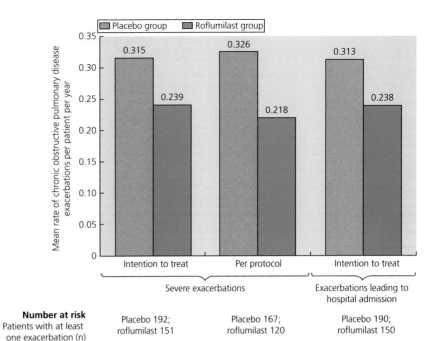

**Figure 16.2** Mean rate of severe exacerbations or exacerbations leading to hospital admission per patient per year. Rate ratios, 95% confidence intervals (CIs) and p values are based on a negative binomial regression model excluding a correction for overdispersion. Reproduced with permission from Martinez et al. (2015).

**Number at risk**
Patients with at least one exacerbation (n)
Rate ratio (95% CI)
Two-sided p value

| Severe exacerbations | | Exacerbations leading to hospital admission |
| --- | --- | --- |
| Placebo 192; roflumilast 151 | Placebo 167; roflumilast 120 | Placebo 190; roflumilast 150 |
| 0.757 (0.601–0.952) | 0.668 (0.518–0.861) | 0.761 (0.604–0.960) |
| 0.0175 | 0.0018 | 0.0209 |

---

Box 16.3 **Novel anti-inflammatory treatments for COPD.**

- Phosphodiesterase-4 inhibitors (e.g. roflumilast)
- p38 Mitogen-activated protein kinase inhibitors (e.g. SB-681323)
- Nuclear factor-κB inhibitors (e.g. AS602868)
- Phosphoinositide-3-kinase-γ and -δ inhibitors
- Janus-activated kinase inhibitors
- Peroxisome proliferator-activated receptor-γ agonists (e.g. rosiglitazone)
- Adhesion molecule inhibitors (e.g. bimosiamose)
- Non-antibiotic macrolides
- Resveratrol analogues

Corticosteroid resistance is one of the typical features of COPD. An alternative therapeutic strategy is therefore to reverse the molecular mechanism of this resistance, which appears to be due to reduced expression and activity of the nuclear enzyme histone deacetylase (HDAC)-2. This can be achieved *in vitro* by theophylline, which acts as an HDAC activator, or by inhibiting oxidative stress. Other therapeutic strategies to reverse steroid resistance include macrolides, nortriptyline and phosphoinositide-3-kinase-δ inhibitors, all of which restore HDAC2 levels (Box 16.4).

Box 16.4 **Reversal of steroid resistance in COPD.**

- Theophylline (HDAC activator)
- Nortriptyline (HDAC activator)
- Phosphoinositide-3-kinase-δ inhibitors (HDAC activators)
- HDAC2-selective activators
- Antioxidants
- Peroxynitrite scavengers

## Lung repair

Chronic obstructive pulmonary disease is a largely irreversible disease process, but it is possible that enhanced repair of the damage might restore lung function in the future. There has been particular interest in retinoic acid, which is able to reverse experimental emphysema in rats. However, this is unlikely to work in humans, whose lungs do not have the same regenerative capacity; to date, human studies have been negative. Another approach being explored is the use of stem cells in an attempt to regenerate alveolar type 1 cells.

## Route of delivery

Drugs for airway diseases are traditionally given by inhalation. However, inhaler devices usually target larger airways that are predominantly involved in asthma, while elderly patients or those with musculoskeletal problems may have difficulty in using conventional inhaler devices. In COPD, the inflammation is mainly found in the small airways and lung parenchyma, in turn suggesting that devices that deliver drugs more peripherally may be of greater benefit. A more systemic approach facilitated by oral drug delivery is therefore an attractive option, as the lung periphery would be targeted. Oral therapies could also have an impact upon systemic complications that often arise in patients with severe disease, although this would carry an increased risk of adverse effects. An alternative approach is targeted drug delivery by exploiting specific cell uptake mechanisms in target cells, such as macrophages.

## Targeted lung denervation

In COPD, parasympathetic nerves release acetylcholine which in turn causes smooth muscle to contract and mucus production, both of which lead to airway obstruction and symptoms. Targeted lung denervation is a novel bronchoscopic therapy that ablates the parasympathetic innervation surrounding the main bronchi, and may have a similar mechanism of action to that of anticholinergic drugs. Preliminary data have indicated some benefit from this technique, although whether it will confer meaningful long-term benefit requires further analysis.

## Further reading

Barnes PJ. Corticosteroid resistance in patients with asthma and chronic obstructive pulmonary disease. *Journal of Allergy and Clinical Immunology* 2013; **131**: 636–645.

Barnes PJ. New anti-inflammatory treatments for chronic obstructive pulmonary disease. *Nature Reviews Drug Discovery* 2013; **12**: 543–559.

Barnes PJ. Identifying molecular targets for new drug development for chronic obstructive pulmonary disease: What does the future hold? *Seminars in Respiratory and Critical Care Medicine* 2015; **36**: 508–522.

Cazzola M, Matera MG. Bronchodilators: current and future. *Clinics in Chest Medicine* 2014; **35**: 191–201.

Martinez FJ, Calverley PM, Goehring UM, Brose M, Fabbri LM, Rabe KF. Effect of roflumilast on exacerbations in patients with severe chronic obstructive pulmonary disease uncontrolled by combination therapy (REACT): a multi-centre randomised controlled trial. *Lancet* 2015; **385**: 857–966.

Rigotti NA. Smoking cessation in patients with respiratory disease: existing treatments and future directions. *Lancet Respiratory Medicine* 2013; **1**: 241–250.

Singh D. New combination bronchodilators for COPD: current evidence and future perspectives. *British Journal of Clinical Pharmacology* 2015; **79**: 695–708.

Slebos DJ, Klooster K, Koegelenberg CFN et al. Targeted lung denervation for moderate to severe COPD: a pilot study. *Thorax* 2015; **70**: 411–419.

# Index

*ABC of COPD*, Third Edition. Edited by Graeme P. Currie.
© 2017 John Wiley & Sons Ltd. Published 2017 by John Wiley & Sons Ltd.